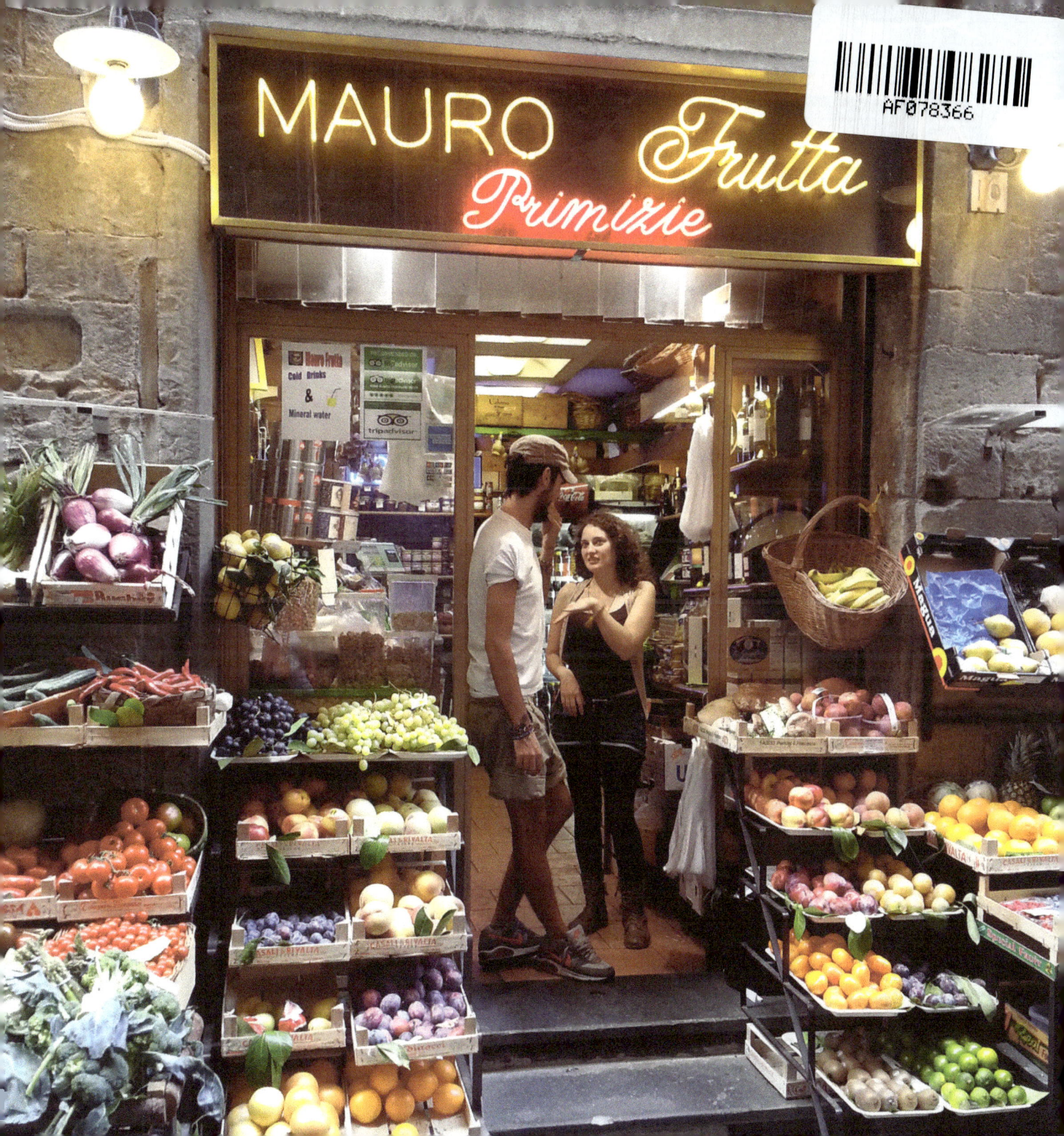

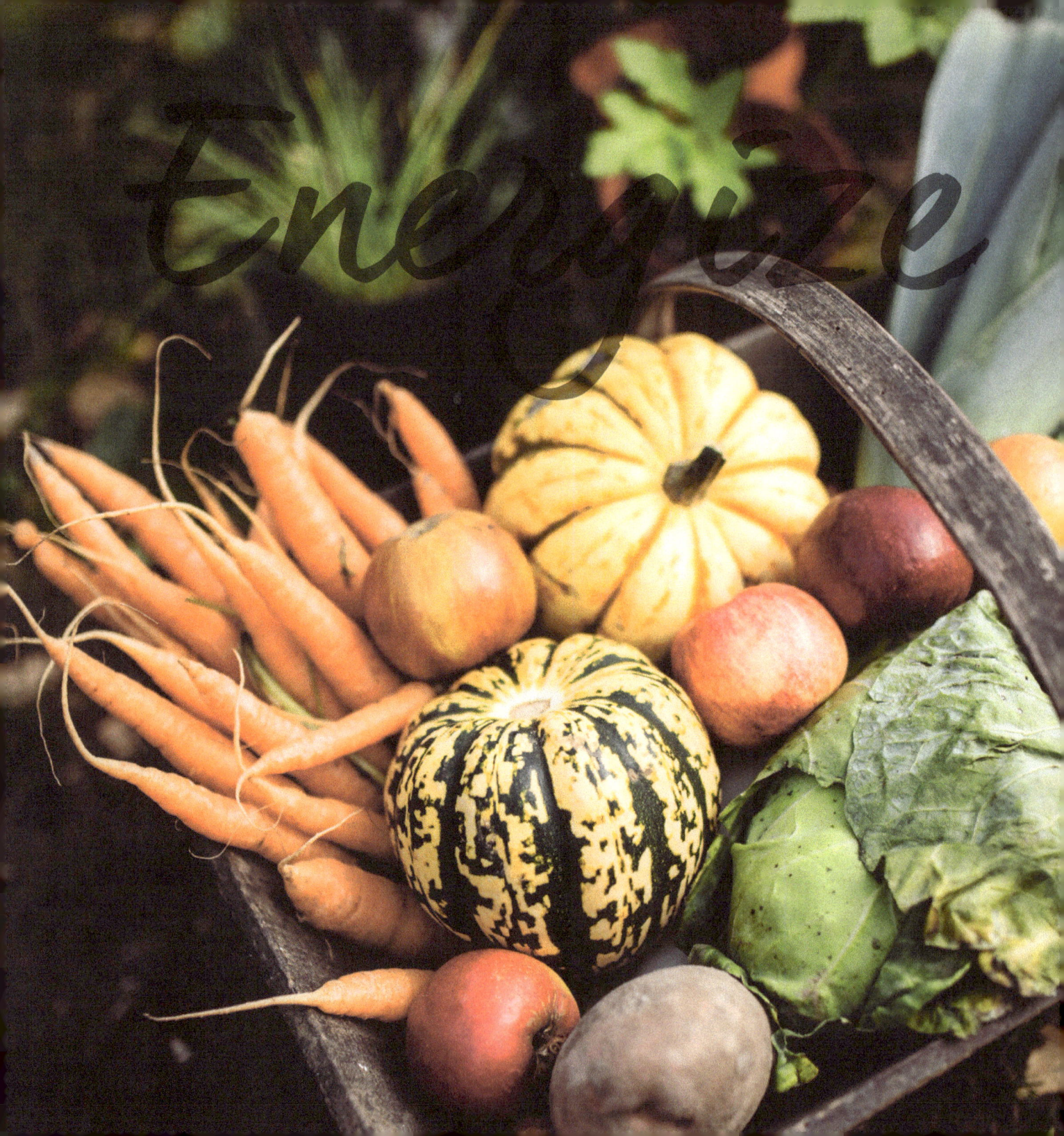

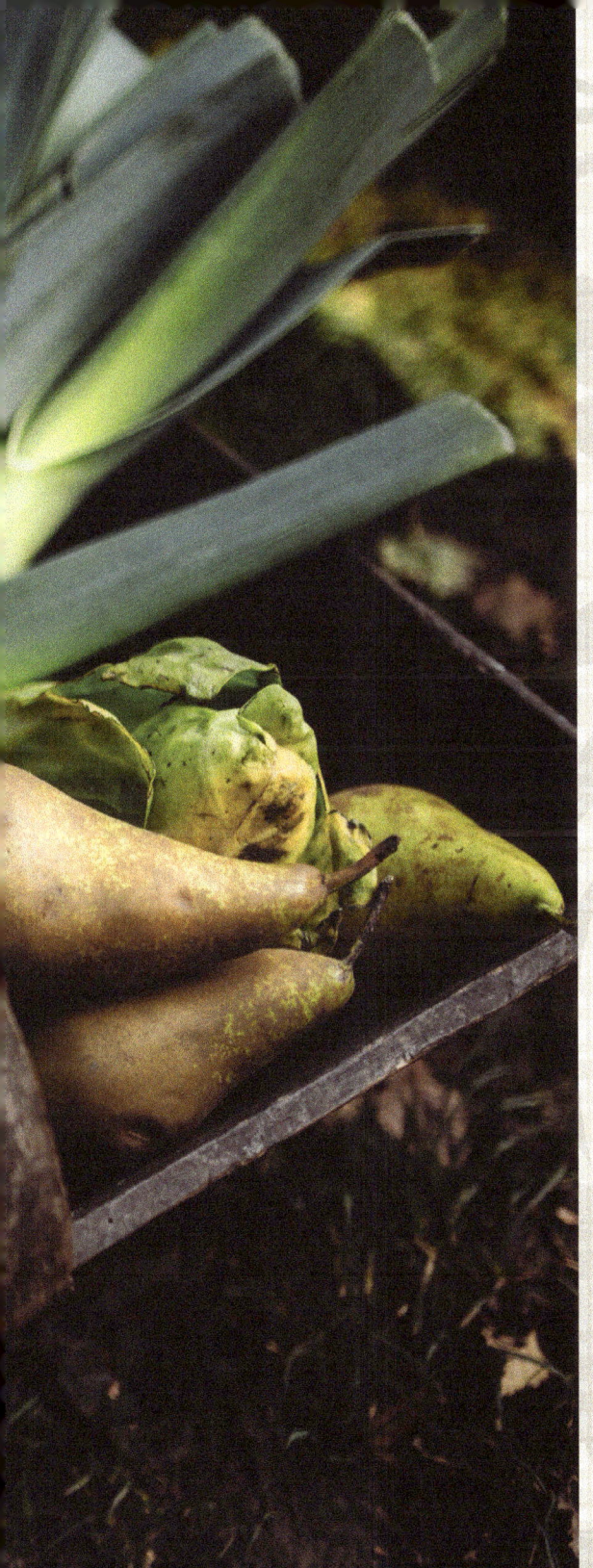

Energize Me superfoods

Nutrient Dense Whole foods,
Grain Free and Dairy Free Recipes

Deb Pozingis

Copyright @ 2015 Deb Pozingis
Photography 2015 Deb Pozingis
Front cover Design Deb Pozingis and Leigh Fabian
Graphic Design Leigh Fabian

All rights reserved. No part of this publication may be reproduced or distributed in any other form or by any means, electronic or mechanical, or stored in a database or retrieval system, without prior written permission from the publisher and the author.

The author of this book does not dispense medical advice or prescribe the use of any technique as a form of treatment for physical, emotional, or medical problems without the advice of a physician, either directly or indirectly. The intent of the author is only to offer information of a general nature to help you in your quest for emotional and spiritual well-being. In the event you use any information in this book for yourself, which is your constitutional right, the author and the publisher assume no responsibility in any manner for any adverse effects arising from your actions.

National Library of Australia Cataloguing-in-Publication entry

Creator: Pozingis, Deb, author.
Title: Energize me superfoods : grain free & dairy free recipes /Deb Pozingis (author) ;
graphic design by L. Fabian.
Edition: 1st ed.
ISBN: 9780994159700 (paperback)
ISBN: 9780994159724 (ebook)
Subjects: Food allergy--Diet therapy--Recipes.Milk-free diet--Recipes.
Other Creators/Contributors: Fabian, L., designer.
Dewey Number: 641.56318
Edition: 1st ed.

Whole foods, Dairy Free, Grain Free, Raw, Gluten Free recipes
2nd Edition February 2015
www.energizemefc.com

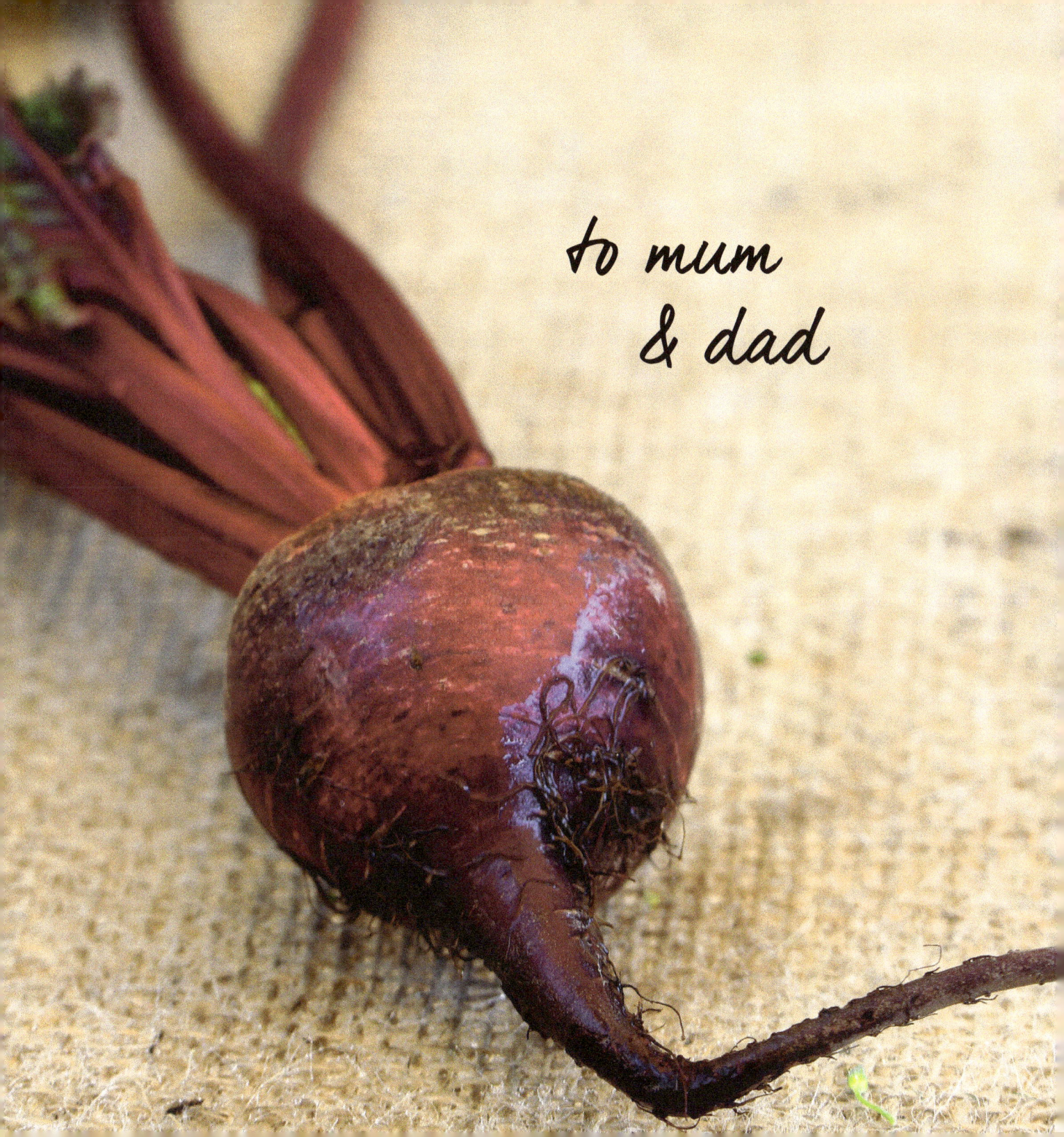

Acknowledgements:

To my family and friends I thank you, especially for putting up with me and enduring each of my new cooking fads over the years. Thank you to my two beautiful sons Reece & Pierce that had no option but to eat my food growing up. I love you for that and without your honest feedback this book would not be where it is today and I value your input. I thank you for your encouragement and support.

A special thank you to my loving parents Joan and Peter for empowering me through this statement
"You can achieve anything you want in this life, there is nothing stopping you if you set your mind to it".

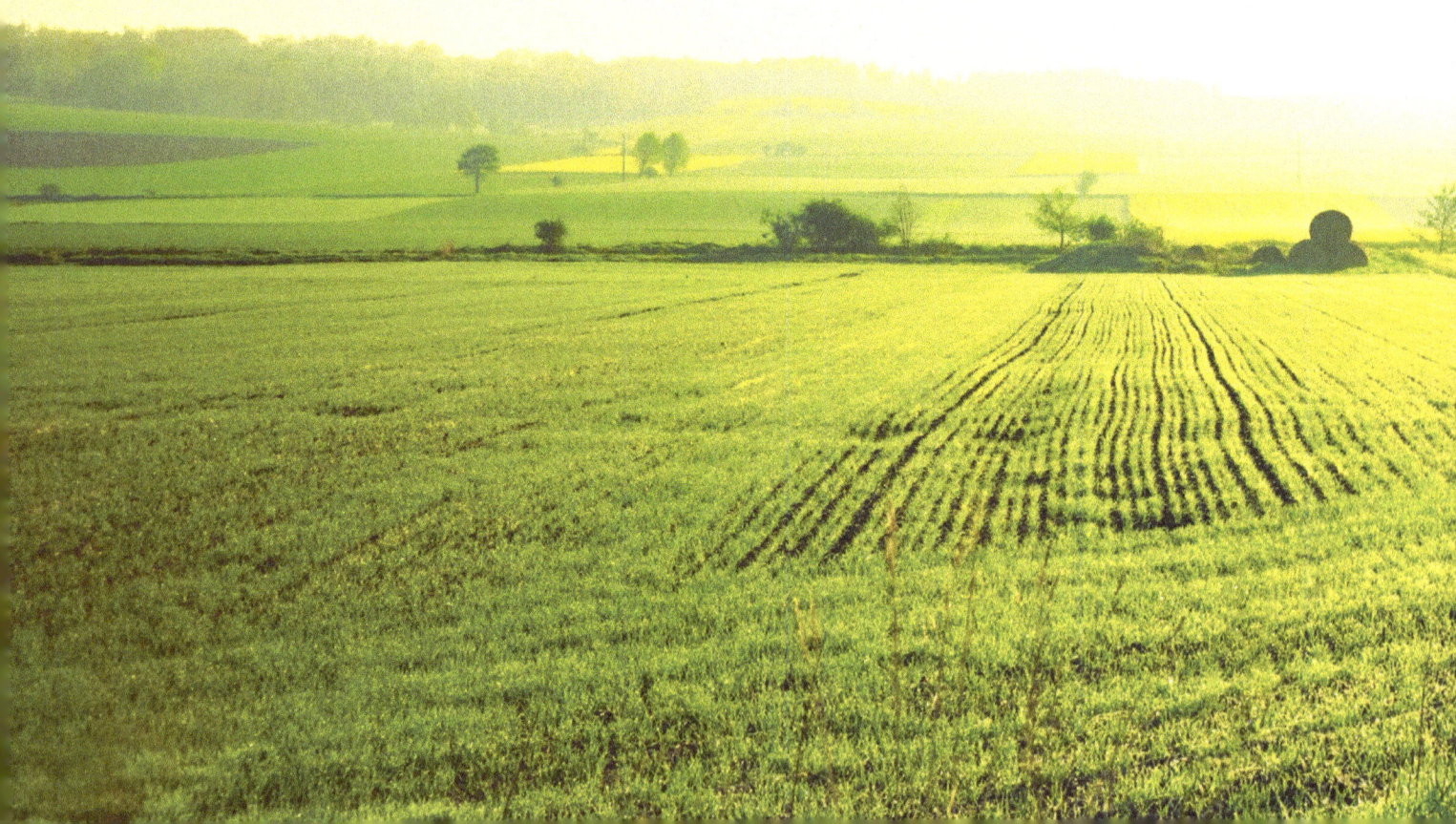

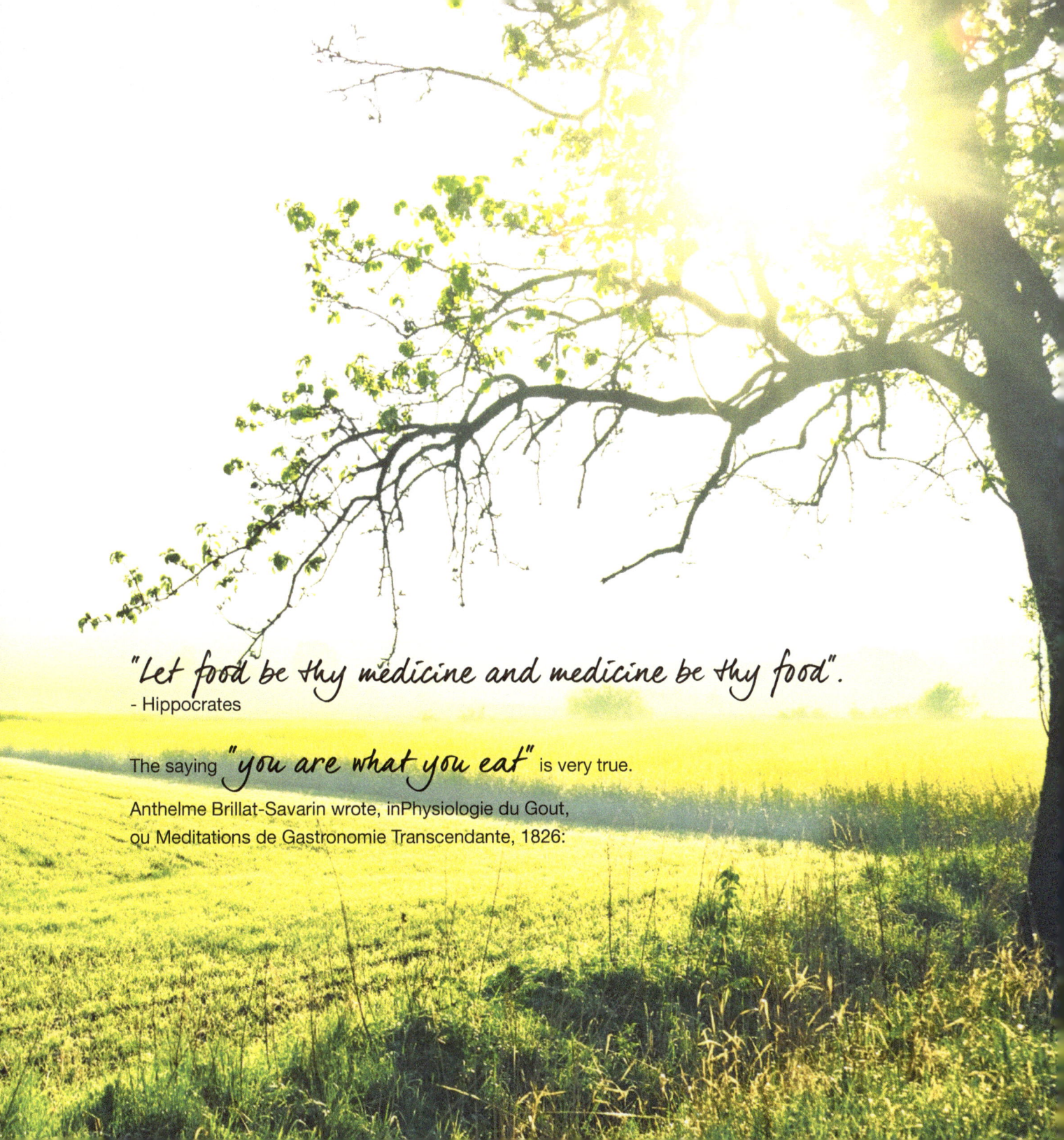

"Let food be thy medicine and medicine be thy food".
- Hippocrates

The saying "you are what you eat" is very true.

Anthelme Brillat-Savarin wrote, in Physiologie du Gout,
ou Meditations de Gastronomie Transcendante, 1826:

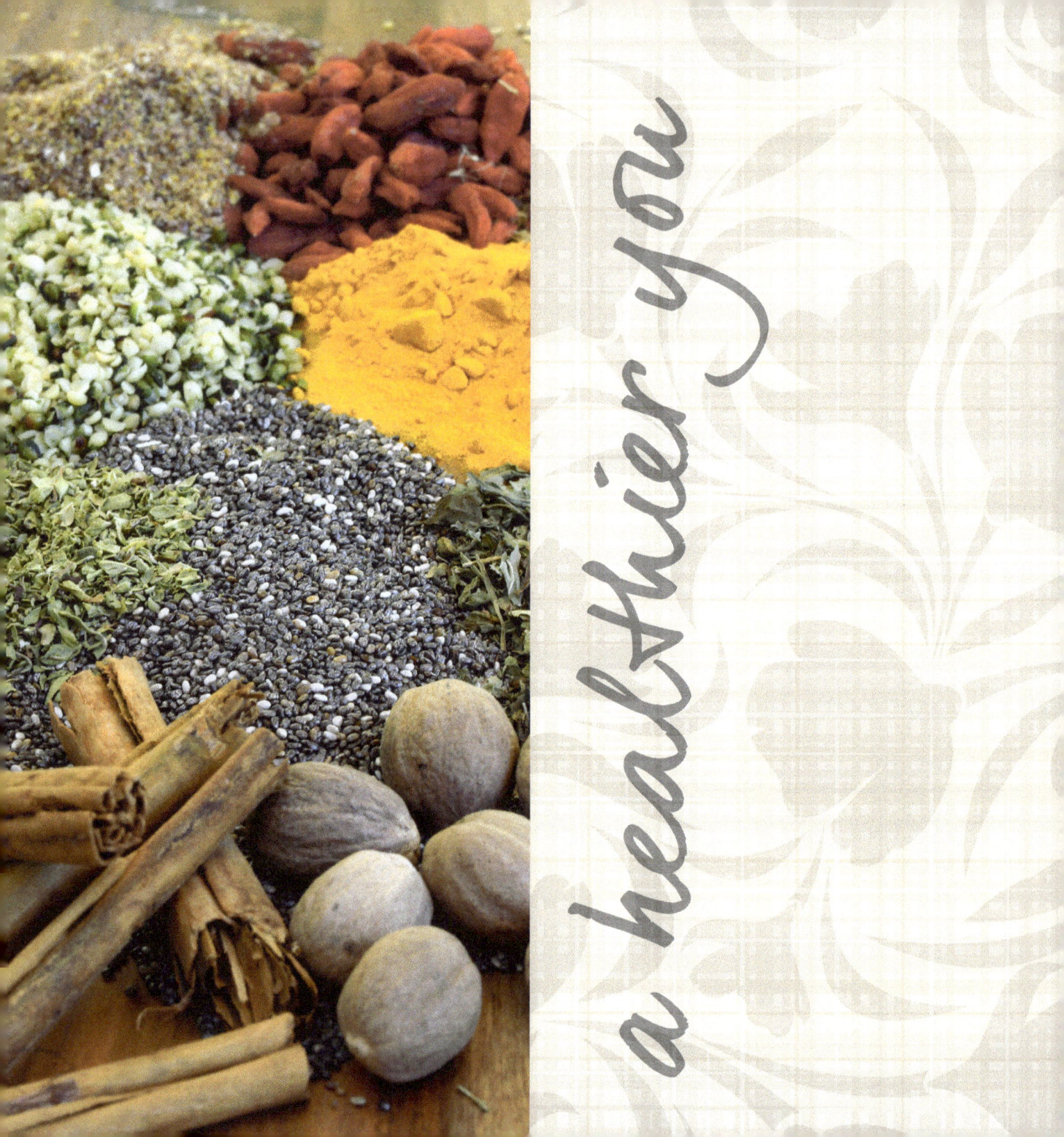

a healthier you

Intro

Are you sick of feeling tired, bloated or lacking energy on a daily basis? Do you often suffer from feeling sleepy midafternoon most days? Did you know that the food you are eating could be the major cause of this?

Most people do not realize the direct relationship between the food they eat and how it makes their body feel and function. The body responds differently to each and everything we eat. This is not a fad diet book; there are no counting calories or any secret tonics or elixirs.

Everyone I have coached and educated over the years, including my own self-discovery with food, have watched the excess weight simply disappear by eating the types of foods in this book. By getting back to the basics, eating whole foods, I now eat whenever I am hungry without the worry of counting calories or putting on excess weight. The simple and easy recipes in this book will help get you started to a healthier more energized you.

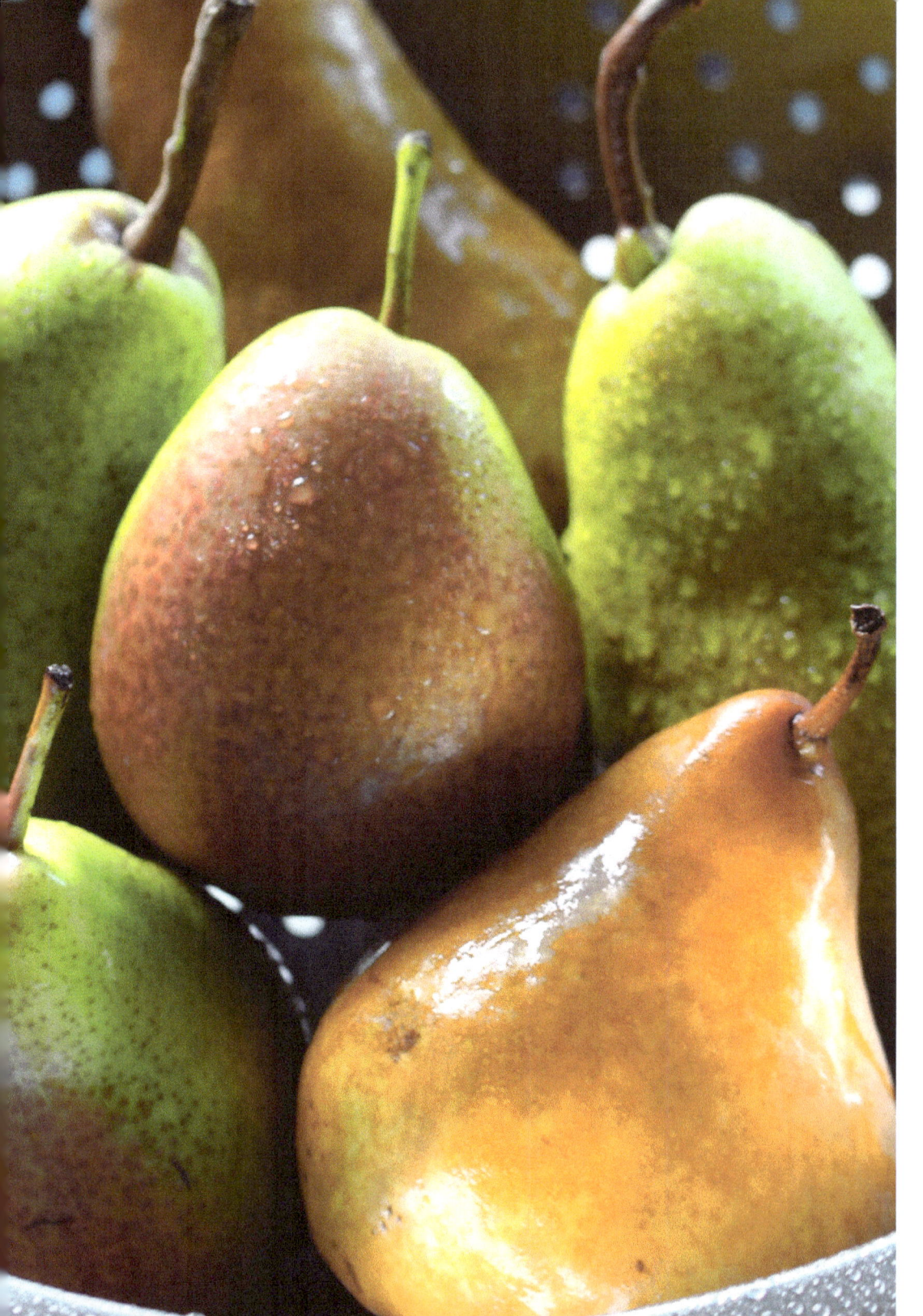

Contents

Smoothies & Juices

1. Berry fruit smoothie
2. Orange pine smoothie
3. Choc-berry smoothie
4. Super green smoothie
5. Chocolate nut smoothie
6. Pear & cinnamon smoothie
7. Banana coconut smoothie
8. Breakfast detox juice
9. Apple celery carrot juice
10. Green tea- spinach-mint

Infused Waters

1. Refreshing berry water
2. Lemon cucumber water
3. Green tea with lemon and mint water

Breakfast

1. Grain free muesli
2. Grain free pancakes
3. High protein salmon omelet
4. Breakfast omelet
5. Beef strips with egg and spinach
6. Poached eggs on sweet potato hash brown

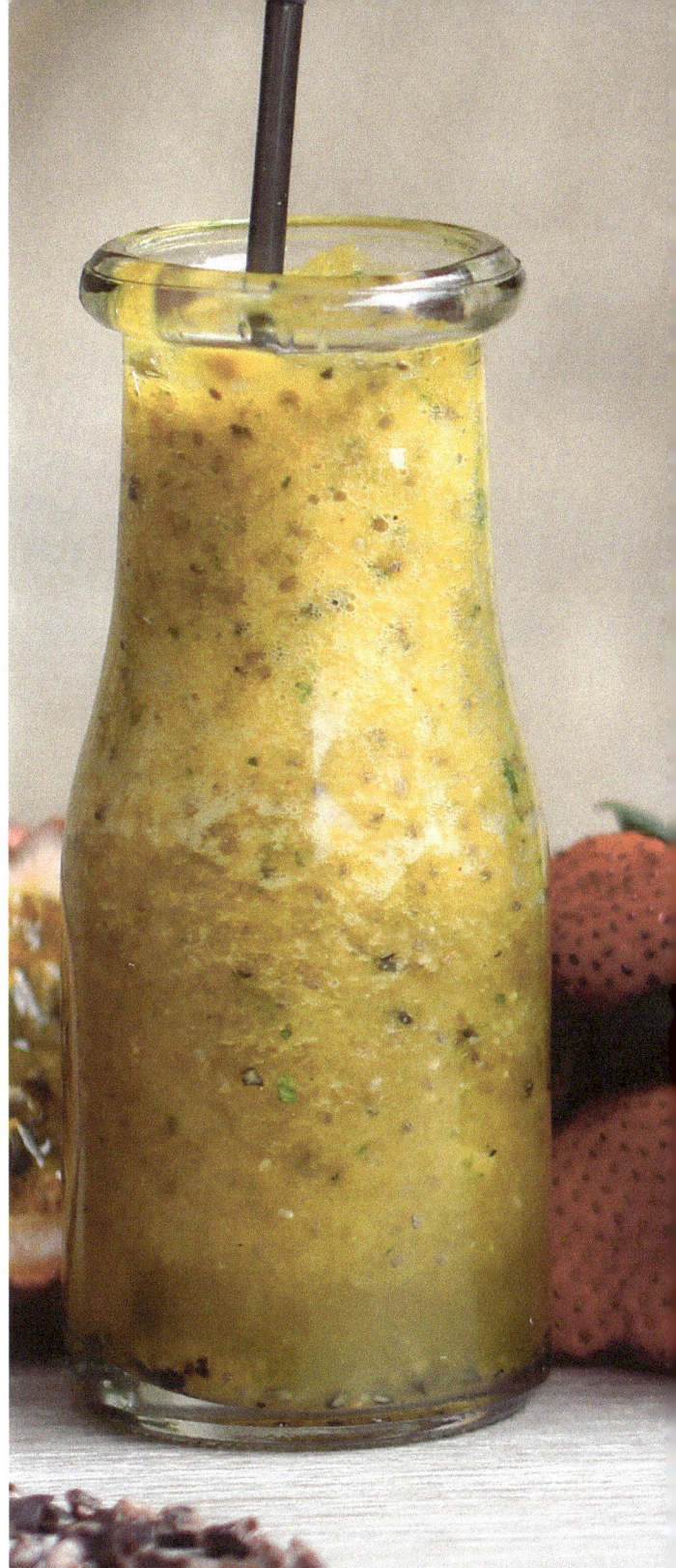

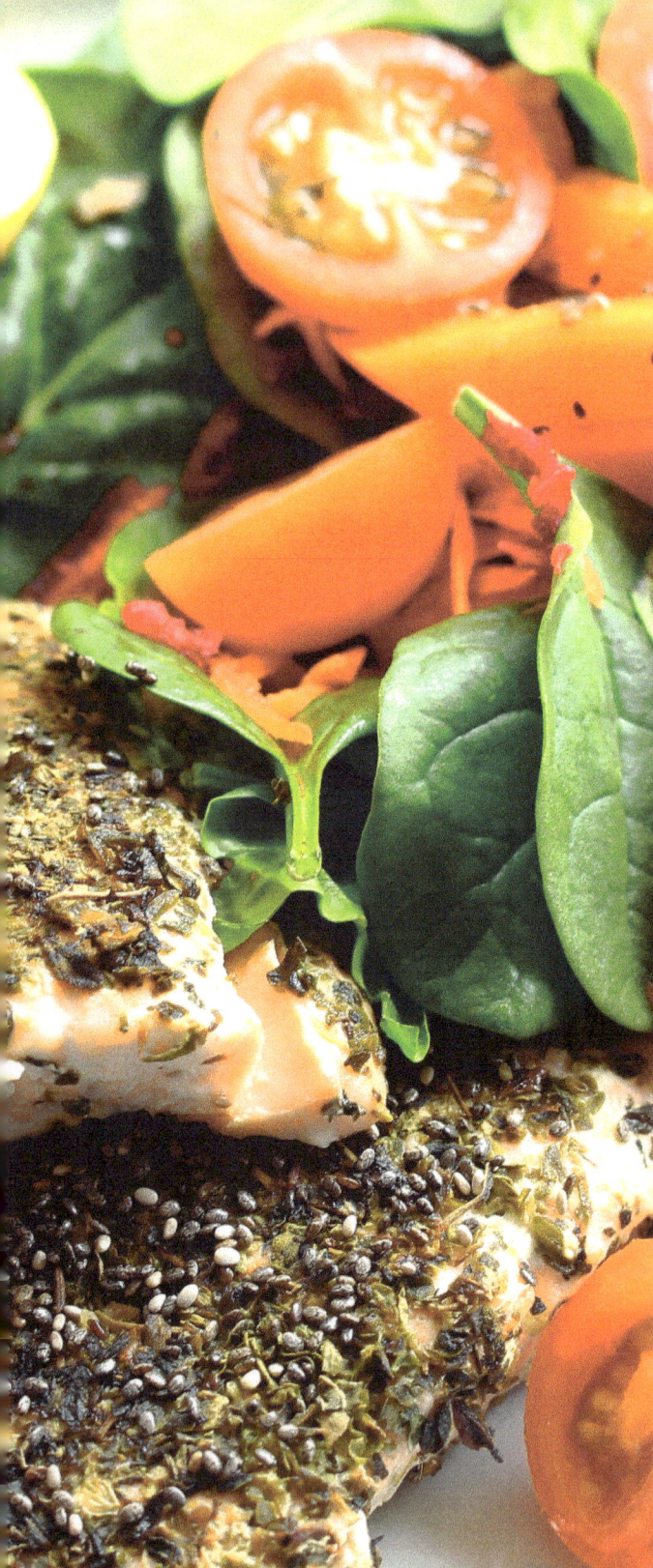

Dips & Crisps

1. Spicy avocado dip
2. Beetroot dip
3. Creamy tahini dip
4. Tangy tomato salsa dip
5. Salmon dip
6. Sesame seed baked crisps

Soups

1. Pumpkin soup
2. Tomato soup
3. Vegetable soup
4. Lamb & pumpkin soup
5. Spicy thai soup
6. Broccoli spinach soup

Dinner

1. Atlantic salmon & salad
2. Prawns on zucchini pasta
3. Roasted chicken breast on cauliflower puree'
4. Beef / chicken strips with tomato and spinach
5. Chicken or Lamb curry
6. Homemade pizza base (grain free) plus toppings
7. Ground beef burgers
8. Sauté chicken Kebabs
9. Spicy chicken kebabs
10. Beef Cabbage rolls
11. Roast lamb and Mediterranean vegetables
12. Vegetable spinach lasagna
13. Mushroom and tomato frittata

Side Vegetables

1. Baked sweet potato wedges
2. Baked carrots
3. Baked zucchini
4. Steamed vegetables
5. Baked Mediterranean vegetables

Salads

1. Greek salad
2. Raw beetroot & carrot salad
3. Pear/Apple & almond salad
4. Spring salad
5. Asian salad
6. Chia mixed salad

Salad Dressings

1. Creamy capsicum salad dressing
2. Mustard-orange garlic salad dressing
3. Lemon-herb dressing
4. Apple cider vinegar vinaigrette
5. Spicy tomato sauce
6. Creamy saute sauce

Fermented Vegies

1. Sauerkraut
2. Cucumbers & peppers
3. Fermented Coconut Cream

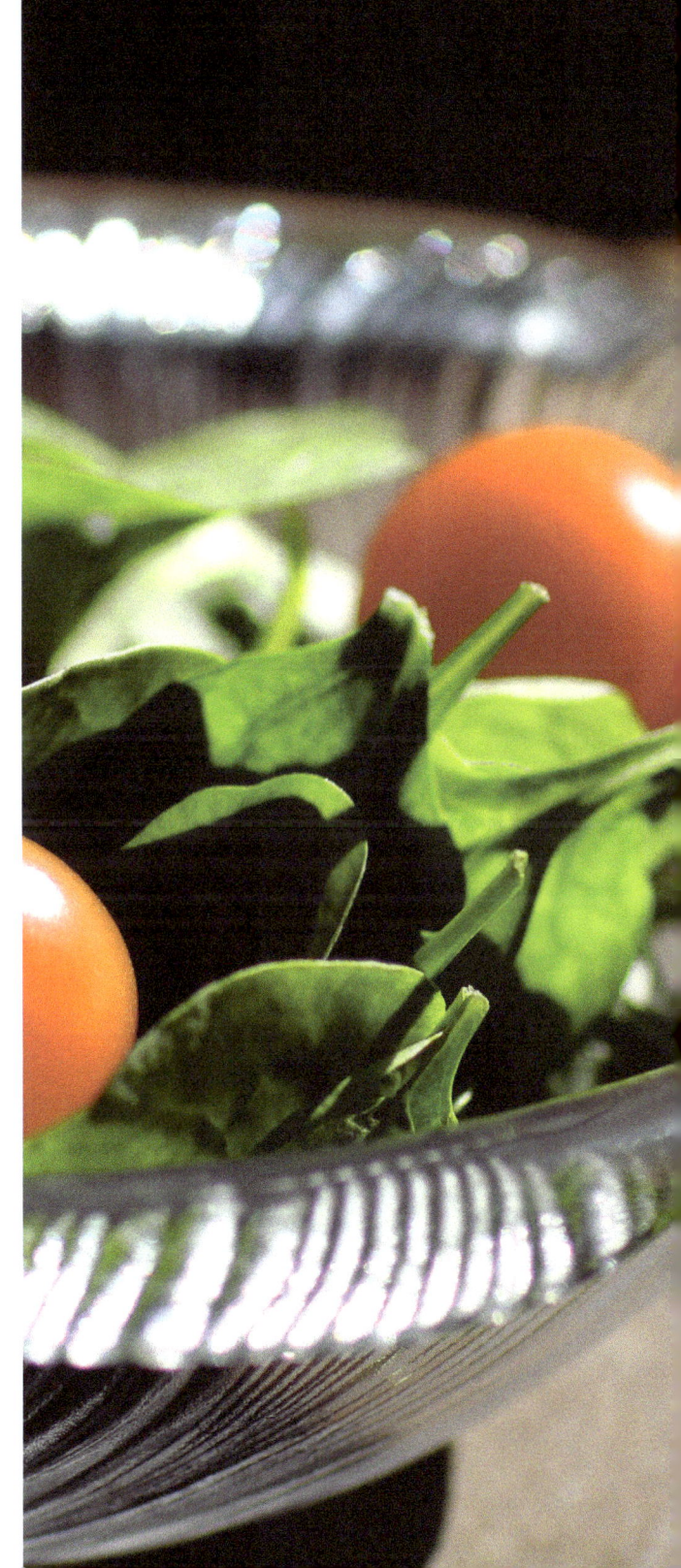

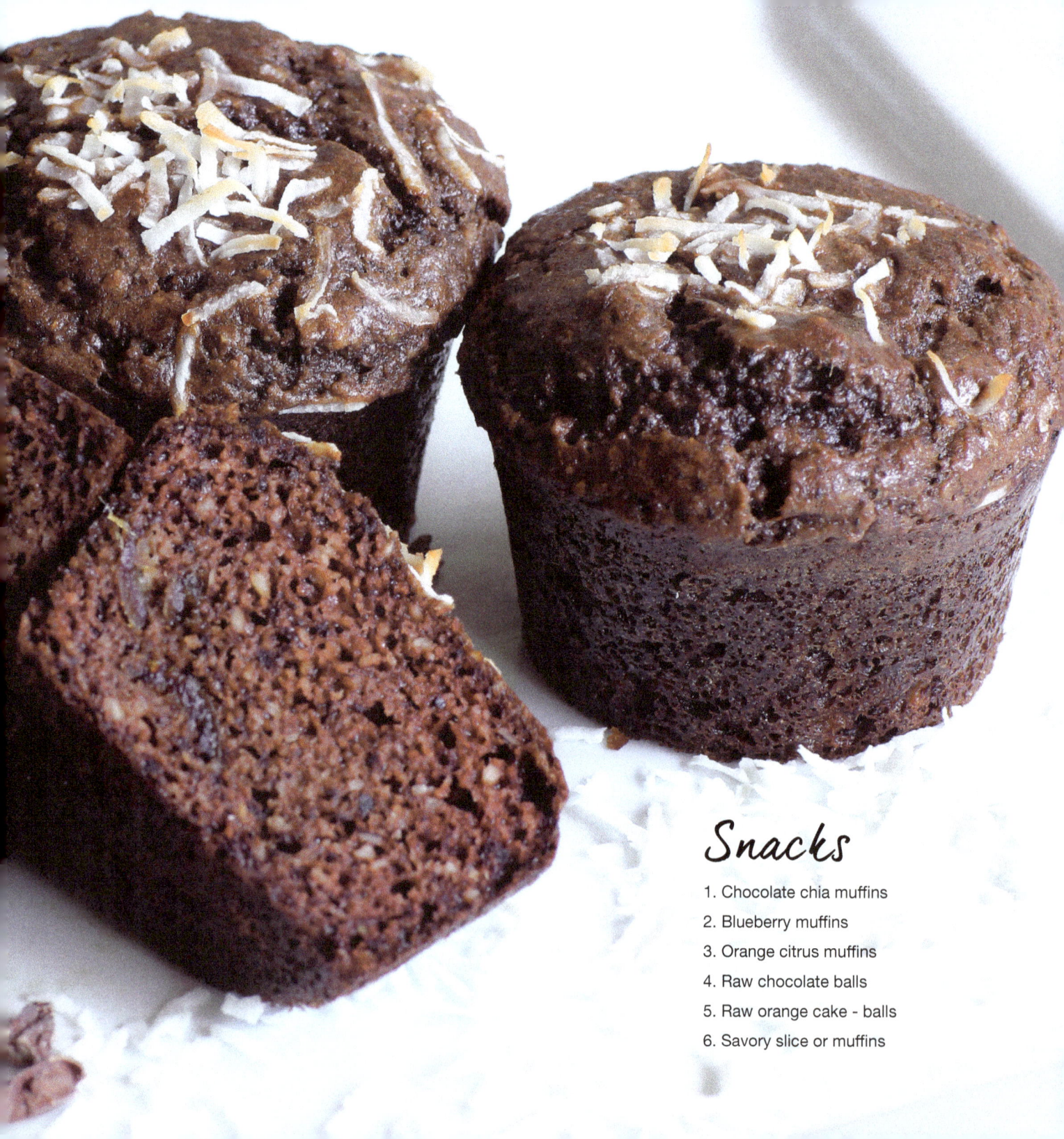

Snacks

1. Chocolate chia muffins
2. Blueberry muffins
3. Orange citrus muffins
4. Raw chocolate balls
5. Raw orange cake - balls
6. Savory slice or muffins

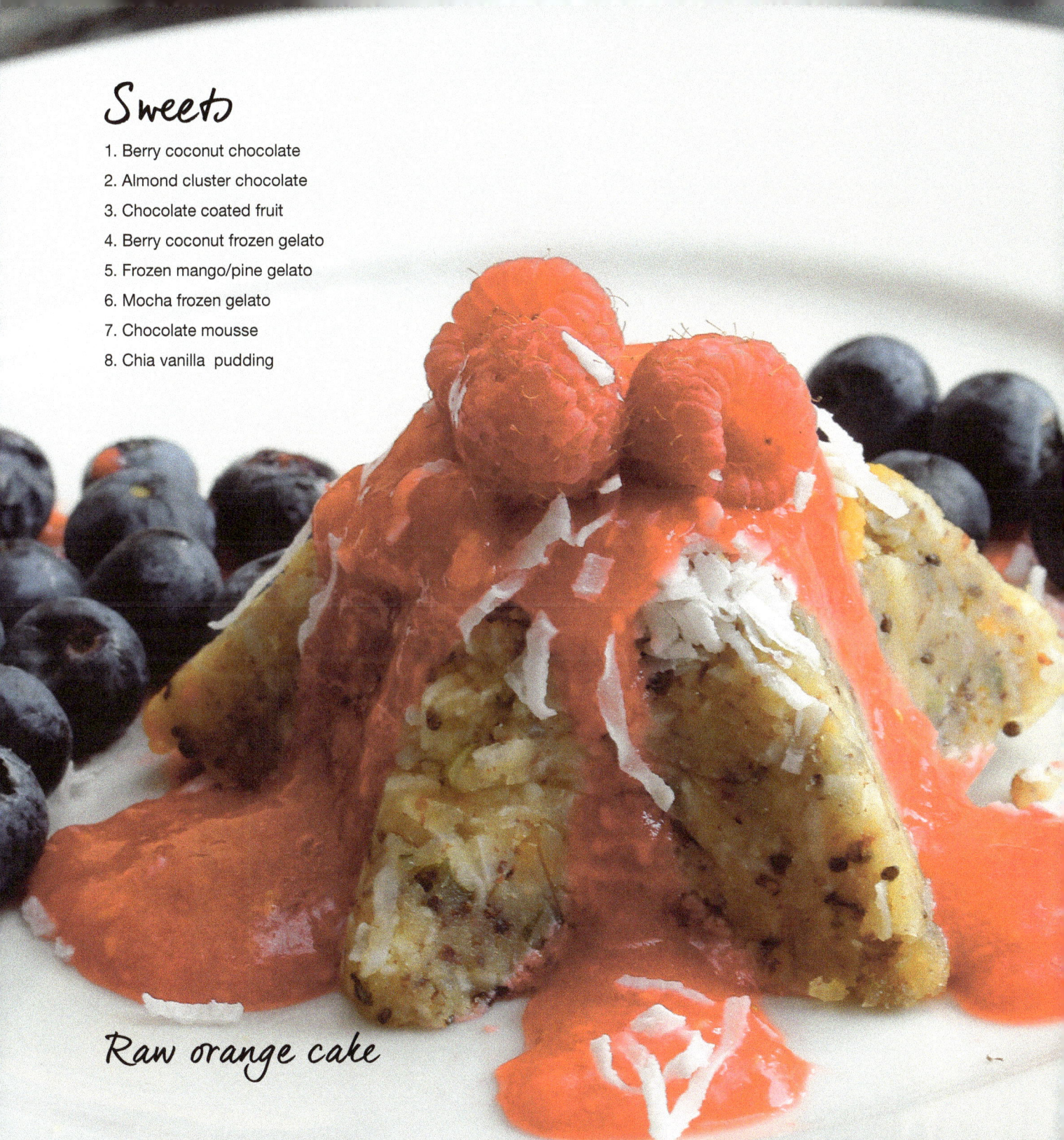

Sweets

1. Berry coconut chocolate
2. Almond cluster chocolate
3. Chocolate coated fruit
4. Berry coconut frozen gelato
5. Frozen mango/pine gelato
6. Mocha frozen gelato
7. Chocolate mousse
8. Chia vanilla pudding

Raw orange cake

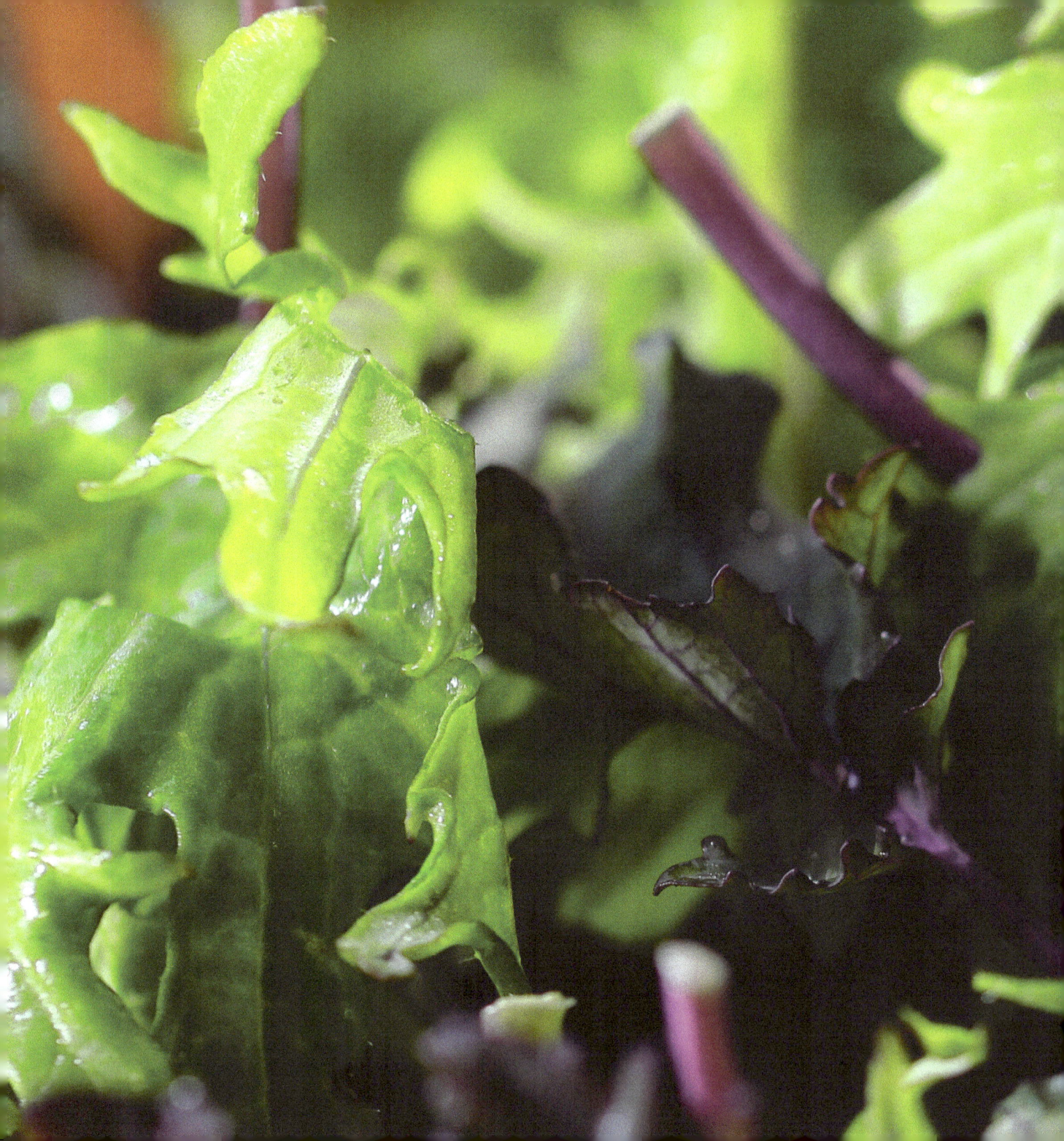

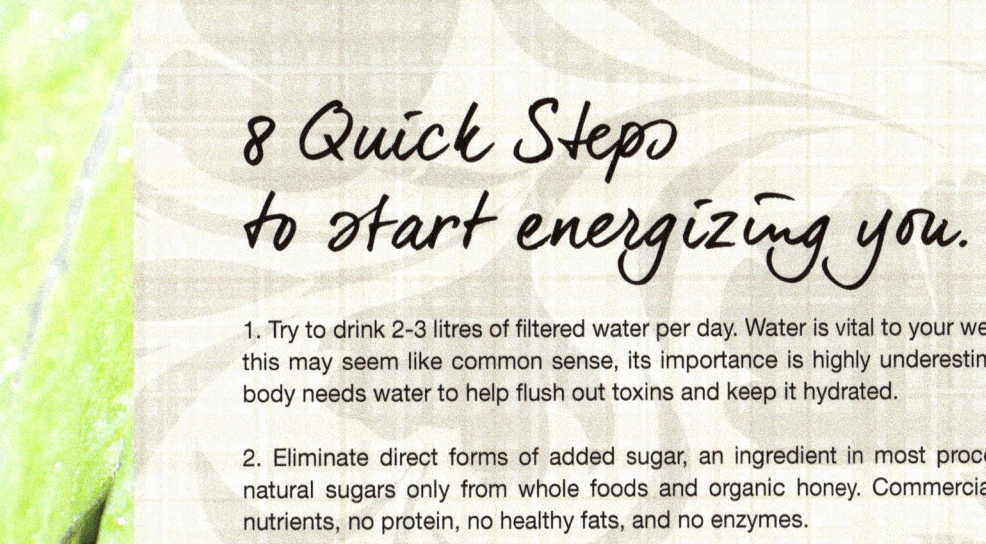

8 Quick Steps to start energizing you.

1. Try to drink 2-3 litres of filtered water per day. Water is vital to your wellbeing and although this may seem like common sense, its importance is highly underestimated by many. Your body needs water to help flush out toxins and keep it hydrated.

2. Eliminate direct forms of added sugar, an ingredient in most processed foods. Obtain natural sugars only from whole foods and organic honey. Commercial sugar contains no nutrients, no protein, no healthy fats, and no enzymes.

3. Gluten is found in wheat, rye, barley and oats. Include few, if any grains in your diet if you have any of the below symptoms after eating foods that contain gluten. Grains are acidic and may cause an unhealthy gut in some. Eating foods that contain grains such as pasta, bread, pastries and cakes may cause symptoms such as bloating, chronic fatigue, nutritional deficiencies, anemia, skin rashes and more.

4. Eating dairy for some people may result in the undigested lactose sitting in their large intestine which is then fermented by natural gut bacteria and causes excessive gas symptoms which include, but are not limited to; bloating, pain or cramps and rumbling sounds in the stomach. If you experience any of these symptoms limiting your dairy intake could be beneficial.

5. Include raw and fermented foods in your diet. Raw food has higher levels of fibre, vitamins, nutrients and living enzymes to feed and repair your body. Buy organic when you can as it has the highest nutrient levels and less damaging chemicals, pesticides and sprays. Introducing fermented foods can help to keep your gut healthy as they contain probiotics in the form of good bacteria.

6. Introduce coconut oil to your diet. Coconut contains lauric acid which may help to protect your body from viral and bacterial infections. Coconut contains omega-3 fats which are important for brain health, stronger teeth and bones. This amazing food contains many beneficial properties, and can be heated to 360 degrees without loss of nutrients.

7. Exercise regularly. Daily exercise, including deep breathing, will help release toxins from your body and stimulate your hormone production into achieving a healthier balance. Try to get out in the fresh air and natural sunlight daily for added doses of vitamin D.

8. Eat lots of food that contains an Alkaline ph level. Studies* are now showing that an alkaline based diet benefits health. By eating predominately alkaline foods there is less stress on the body to maintain a healthy ph level.

*J Environ Public Health. 2012; 2012: 727630. Published online Oct 12, 2011. http://www.ncbi.nlm.nih.gov/pmc/articles/PMC3195546/

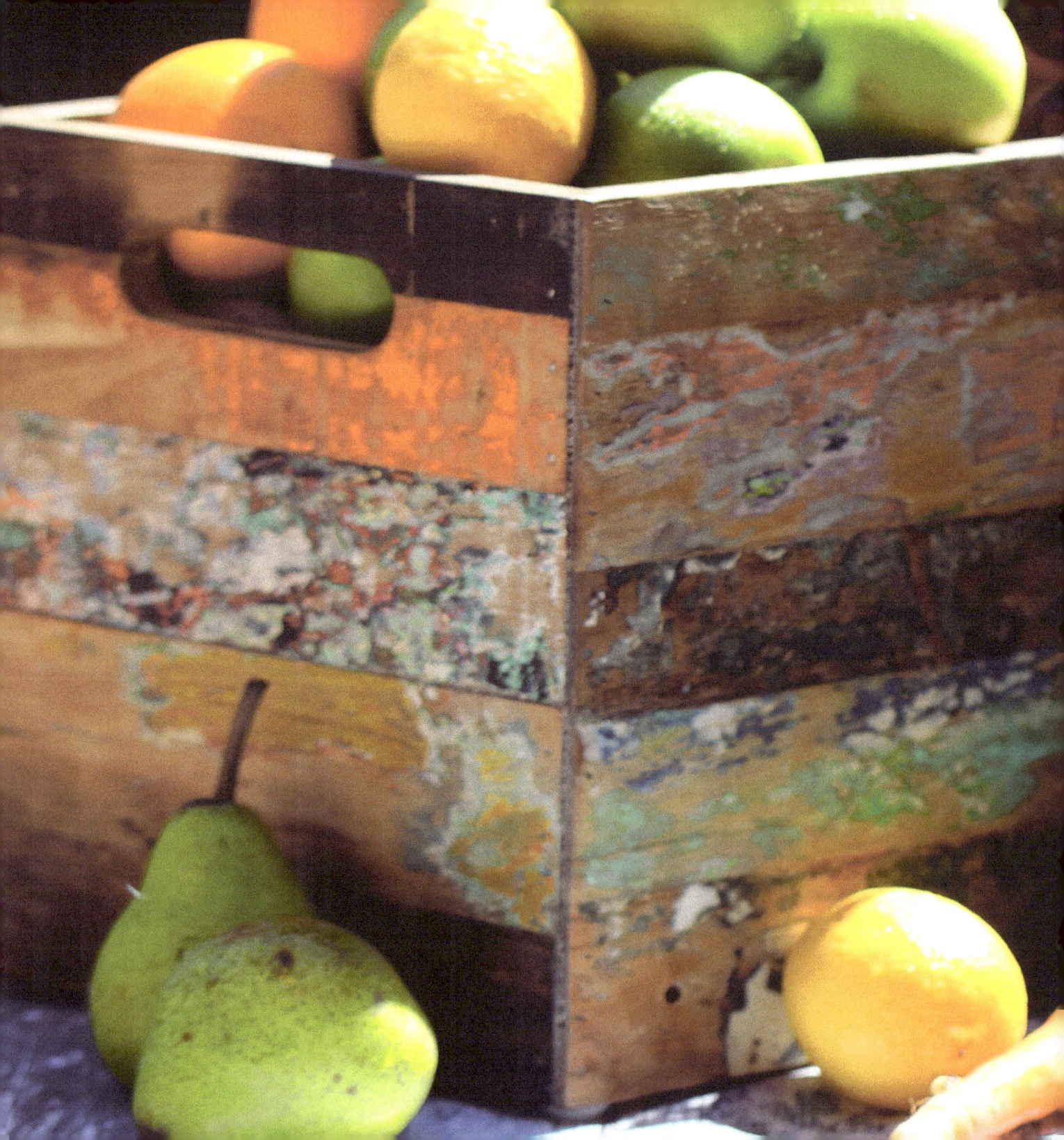

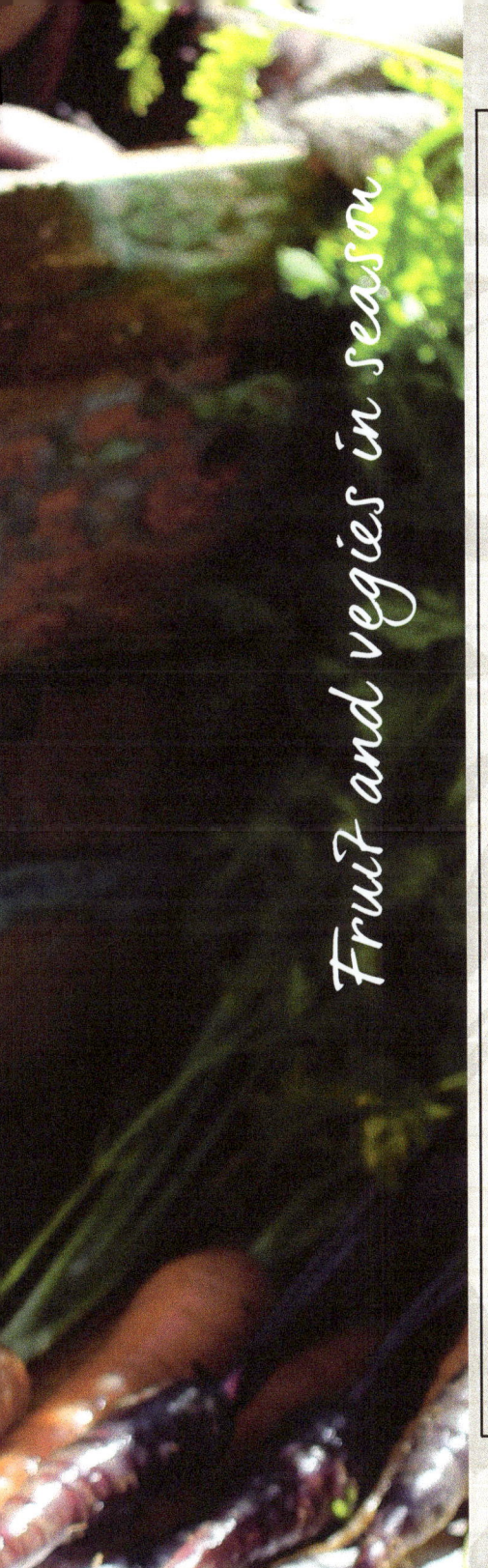

Fruit and vegies in season

Spring	Summer	Autumn	Winter
Apricot	Apricots	Apples	Apples
Avocado	Avocado	Avocado	Avocado
Bananas	Bananas	Bananas	Bananas
Berries	Berries	Figs	Grapefruit
Cherry	Cherries	Grapefruit	Guava
Grapefruit	Figs	Grapes	Kiwifruit
Guava	Grapefruit	Guava	Lemons
lemons	Grapes	Kiwifruit	Limes
Limes	Melons	Lemons	Mandarin
Mandarin	Nectarine	Limes	Oranges (Navel)
Mango	Oranges (Valencia)	Mandarins (Imperial)	Pears
Melons	Passion fruit	Mango	Passion fruit
Nectarine	Pineapple	Melons	Pineapple
Orange	Peaches	Nectarine	Quince
Passion fruit	Pears	Oranges (Valencia)	Tangelo
Papaya	Plums	Papaya	Strawberry
Pineapple	Strawberries	Passion fruit	Artichokes (Jerusalem)
Strawberries	Asian Greens	Peach	Asian greens
Artichokes (globe)	Basil	Pears	Broad Beans
Asian greens	Beans	Plum	Beetroot
Asparagus	Beetroot	Pomegranate	Broccoli
Beans	Broccoli	Strawberries	Brussels Sprouts
Broad Beans	Capsicum	Asian greens	Cabbage
Beetroot	Carrots	Beans	Carrots
Broccoli	Celery	Beetroot	Cauliflower
Cabbage	Chillies	Broccoli / Broccolini	Celery
Capsicum	Corn	Brussels Sprouts	Eggplant
Carrots	Cucumber	Cabbage	Fennel
Cauliflower	Eggplant	Capsicum	Kale
Chillies	Leeks	Carrots	Leeks
Cucumber	Lettuce	Cauliflower	Lettuce
Eggplant	Mushroom	Celery	Mushroom
Garlic	Onions	Chillies	Onions
Leeks	Parsley	Corn	Parsley
Lettuce	Peas	cucumber	Parsnips
Mushroom	Potatoes	Eggplant	Peas (snow)
Onions	Radish	Leeks	Potatoes
Parsley	Rhubarb	Lettuce	Rhubarb
Parsnips	Silverbeet	Mushroom	Silverbeet
Peas	Snow peas	Onions	Spinach
Peas (snow)	Spring Onion	Parsley	Spring Onion
Potatoes	Squash	Parsnips	Truffles
Pumpkin	Sweet corn	Peas	Turnips
Radishes	Tomatoes	Potato	Zucchini
Rhubarb	Zucchini	Pumpkin	
Silverbeet		Radishes	
Spinach		Rhubarb	
Spring Onion		Silverbeet	
Squash		Spinach	
Sweetcorn		Spring Onion	
Tomato		Squash	
Zucchini		Sweetcorn	
		Sweet Potatoes	
		Tomatoes	
		Turnip	
		Zucchini	

It is wise to buy fruits and vegetables in season as they more likely to be fresh and supplied by a local producer, not to mention more economical.

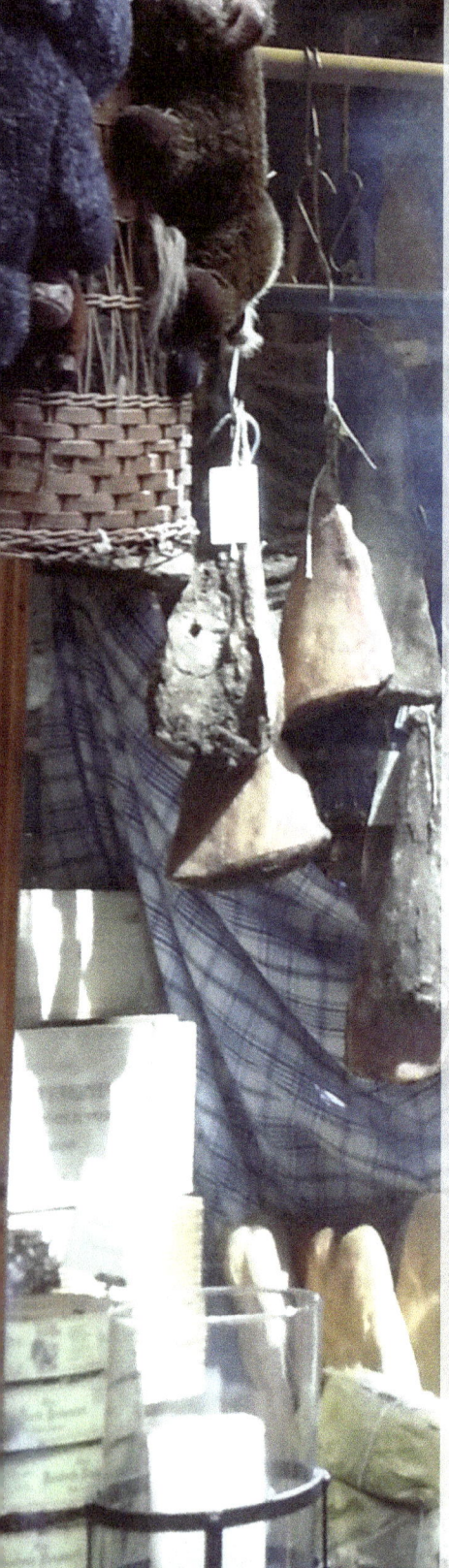

Acidifying Foods

Fats & Oils
- Avocado Oil
- Canola Oil
- Corn Oil
- Flax seed Oil
- Hemp seed Oil
- Lard
- Olive Oil
- Safflower Oil
- Seasame Oil
- Sunflower Oil

Fruits
- Cranberries

Grains
- Barley
- Buckwheat
- Corn Oil
- Hemp Seed Flour
- Kamut
- Oats
- Quinoi
- Rice
- Rye
- Spelt
- Wheat

Dairy
- Butter
- Cheese Cow
- Cheese Goat
- Cheese Processed
- Cheese Sheep
- Milk
- Yoghurt

Nuts & Butters
- Brazil Nuts
- Cashews
- Peanuts
- Pecans
- Tahini
- Walnuts

Animal Protein
- Beef
- Carp
- Clams
- Fish
- Lamb
- Lobster
- Mussels
- Oyster
- Pork
- Rabbit
- Salmon
- Scallops
- Shrimp
- Tuna
- Turkey
- Venison

Other
- Distilled Vinegar
- Potatoes
- Wheat Germ

Alchohol
- Beer
- Hard Liquer
- Spirits
- Wine

Drugs & Chemicals
- Herbicides
- Medicines
- Pesticides

Beans & Legumes
- Almond Milk
- Black Beans
- Chick Peas
- Green Beans
- Kidney Beans
- Lentils
- Lima Beans
- Pinto Beans
- Red Beans
- Rice milk
- Soy Beans
- Soy Milk
- White Beans

Alkalizing Foods

Vegetables
- Alfalfa
- Asparagus
- Barley Grass
- Beets
- Broccoli
- Brussel Sprouts
- Cabbage
- Carrot
- Cauliflour
- Celery
- Chorella
- Collard Greens
- Coconut
- Cucumber
- Danelions
- Dulce
- Edible Flowers
- Eggplant
- Fermented Veggies
- Garlic
- Kale
- Kohlrabi
- Lettuce
- Mushrooms
- Mustard Greens
- Nightshade Veggies
- Onions
- Peas
- Peppers/Capsicum
- Pumpkin
- Rutabaga
- Sea Veggies
- Spirulina
- Sprouts
- Squashes
- Watercress
- Wheat Grass
- Wild Greens

Fruits
- All Berries
- Apple
- Apricot
- Avocado
- Banana
- Cantaloupe
- Cherries
- Currents
- Dates
- Figs
- Grapefruit
- Grapes
- Honeydew Melon
- Lemon
- Lime
- Nectarine
- Orange
- Peach
- Pineapple
- Rock Melon
- Tangerine
- Tomato
- Tropical Fruit
- Water Melon

Protein
- Almonds
- Chestnuts
- Chicken Breast
- Cottage cheese
- Eggs
- Flax seeds
- Millet
- Pumpkin seeds
- Sprouted seeds
- Squash seeds
- Sunflower seeds
- Tempeh (fermented)
- Whey Protein Powder

Other
- Alkaline water
- Apple Cider Vinegar
- Bee Pollen
- Fresh Fruit Juice
- Ginseng Tea
- Green Juices
- Green Tea
- Herbal Tea
- Kombucha
- Mineral Water
- Probiotic Cultures
- Veggie Juices

Sweetners
- Stevia

Spices Seasonings
- All herbs
- Chilli Pepper
- Cinnamon
- Curry
- Ginger
- Miso
- Mustard
- Sea Salt
- Tamari

Oriental vegies
- Daikon
- Dandelion Root
- Kombucha
- Maitake
- Nori
- Reishi
- Shitake
- Umeboshi
- Wakame

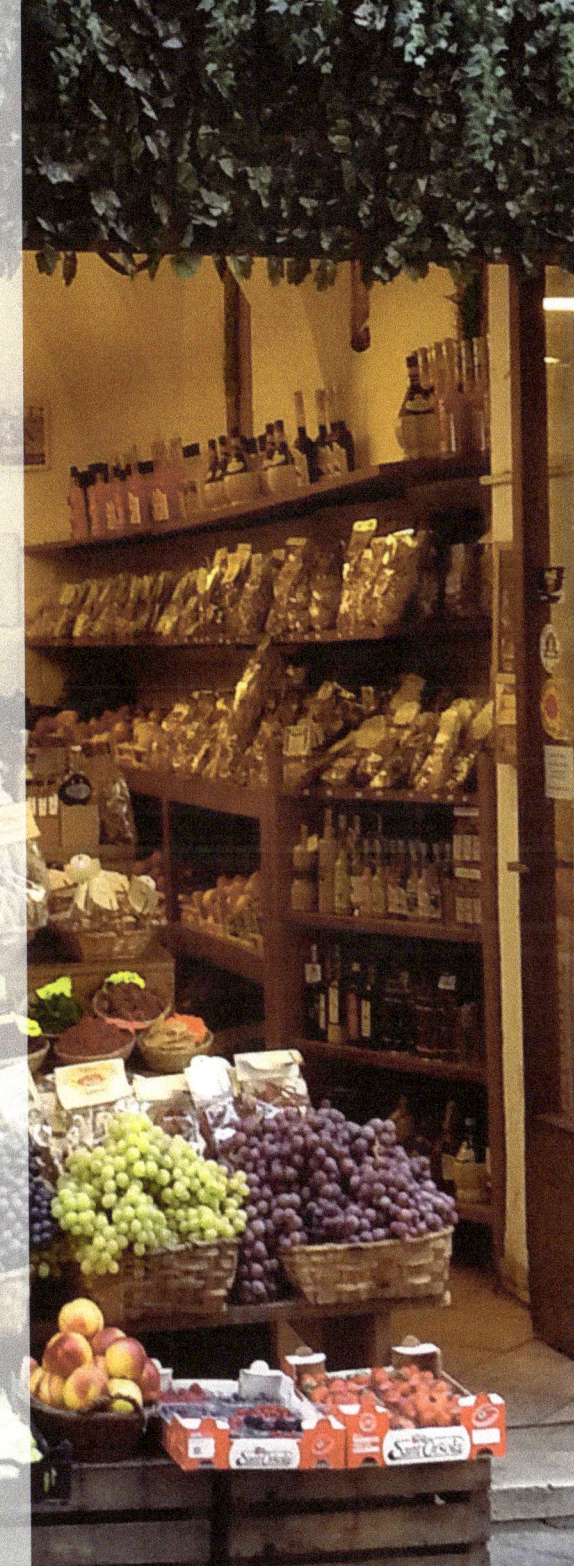

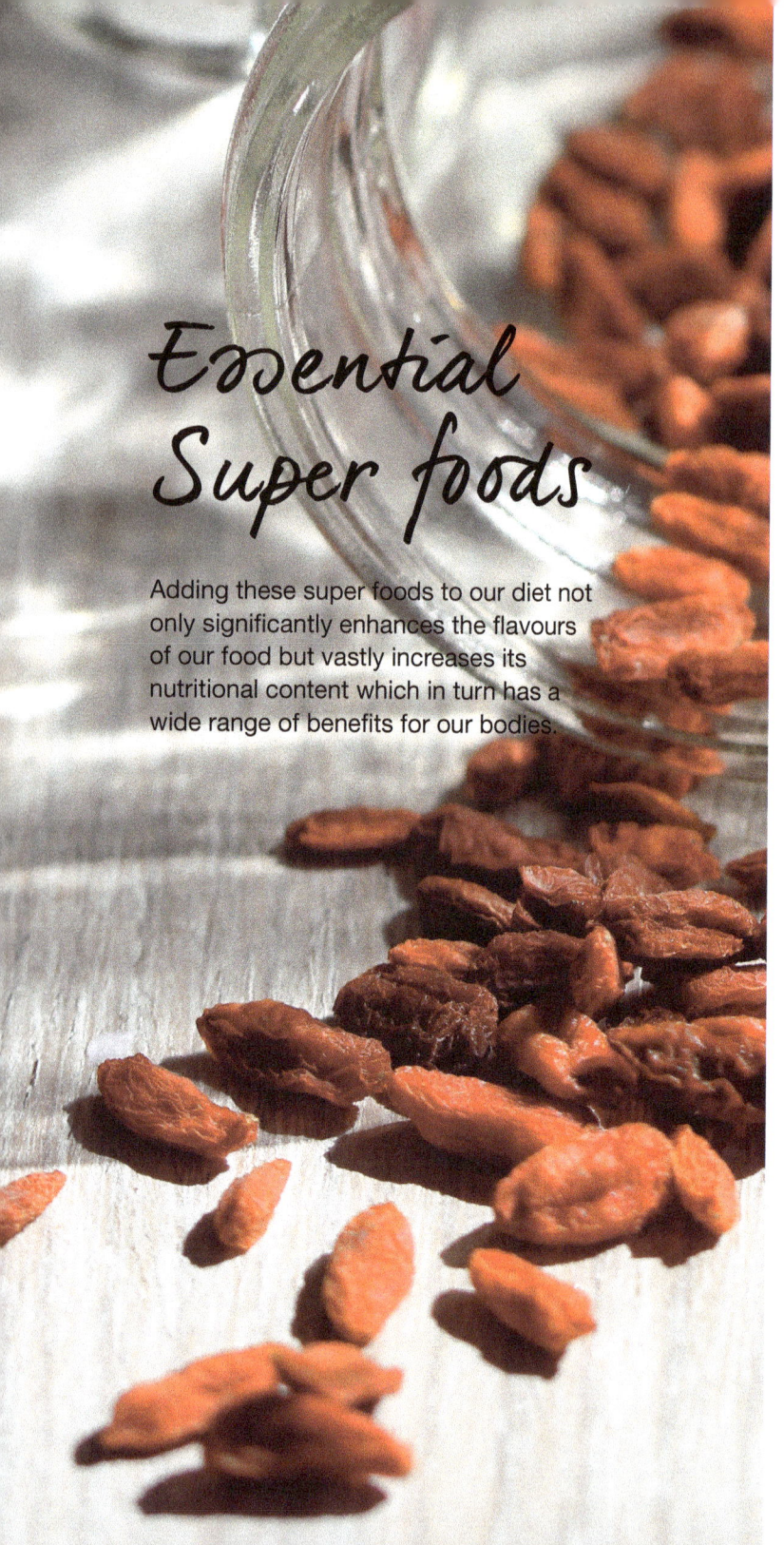

Essential Super foods

Adding these super foods to our diet not only significantly enhances the flavours of our food but vastly increases its nutritional content which in turn has a wide range of benefits for our bodies.

Acai Berry

Açai is absolutely loaded with nutrients. It contains; 19 Amino Acids, Vitamins A, B1, B2, C, E, and P (bioflavonoids), minerals such as potassium, iron, phosphorous, calcium, fibre, trace elements, protein and Omegas 6 and 9 which is unusual for a fruit! Acai berries are very high in antioxidants and assist in fighting free radicals and aging in the body.

Almonds, Cashews, Hazel, & Pine nuts

Nuts in general are known to be healthy and nutritious, containing high-quality protein, lots of healthy fats, vitamins and minerals as well as dietary fibre. They are also dairy and gluten-free.
It is important to eat a variety of nuts as each has its own unique properties.

Cacao

Cacao is one of the richest sources of antioxidants found in nature. It is also a source of important minerals including magnesium and iron. The cacao bean is rich in antioxidants, healthy fats, carbohydrates, protein, polyphenols, minerals like calcium, magnesium, sulfur, copper, iron, zinc and potassium, oleic acid which is a heart-healthy essential monounsaturated fat, fibre and vitamins E, B2, B1, B5, B3 and B9. There are also small amounts of vitamin A and C in raw cacao.

Chia seed

Chia contains calcium, manganese, and phosphorus, its high in fibre and is a great source of healthy omega-3 fats. The unique combination of soluble and insoluble fibre also aid to slow down your body's conversion of starches to sugars, and keeps your body satisfied for longer and less likely to experience "hunger pains". The gelatinous coating chia seeds develop when exposed to liquids can also prevent blood sugar spikes.

Omega-3 fats are important for brain health, stronger teeth and bones and preventing osteoporosis. Manganese is good for your bones and helps your body use other essential nutrients like biotin and thiamine which aid digestion and promotes the health of skin, nails, cells and metabolism. Phosphorus is also used by the body to synthesize protein for cell and tissue growth and repair. Chia seeds also make a great source of protein for vegetarians. Tryptophan is also found in chia seeds, this helps regulate appetite, sleep and improve mood.

Chia Seeds contain 20% Omega-3 Fatty Acids (ALA) (eight times more than salmon), 20% protein with 8 essential amino acids, antioxidants, calcium (five times higher than diary milk), iron (three times more than spinach), Vitamin C (seven times more than oranges) and potassium (double that of a banana).

Coconut

Coconut oil, coconut milk, coconut butter, coconut cream, coconut sugar all comes from the coconut. Coconut research* suggests that by consuming coconut derivatives, it can help prevent heart disease, strokes, dissolve kidney stones, balance blood sugar (control diabetes). They can also enhance the immune system, protect cells against cancer, boost your energy and increases your metabolism. Coconut derivatives can help you shed excess body fat, kill disease-causing bacteria, viruses, and fungi. Furthermore they can relieve symptoms associated with irritable bowel syndrome and protect your skin against free-radical damage that causes premature aging.

*Coconut Research Center. 2010.www.coconutresearchcenter.org

Coconut sugar has a naturally Low Glycemic Index (Low GI) that is nearly half the GI of cane sugar and is also lower than honey. This super food has the added bonus of a nutritional content richer than possibly all other commercially available sweeteners! Coconut sugar contains protein (12 amino acids) and comparatively high mineralization including potassium, magnesium, phosphorous, zinc and iron.

Flaxseed

Flaxseed is one of the sources of essential fatty acids, good for a healthy brain, and anti-inflammatory properties. It is excellent for heart and joint health. Flaxseed is also high in fibre which is good for colon health and your digestive system.

Goji Berries

Goji berries have a cherry-like taste and are a great snack food, packed with 21 minerals, super high in Vitamin C, Vitamin A, containing all of the major Macro nutrients (complete protein (18 amino acids), fat and carbohydrates).

Maca powder

Maca contains numerous minerals and trace elements. It is rich in vitamin B, vitamin C, and E. It provides plenty of calcium, zinc, iron, magnesium, phosphorous and 20+ amino acids. Research shows maca contains compounds that directly support the adrenal glands to help balance hormones and give you energy without being a stimulant. It can help decrease anxiety and stress.

Maqui Berry

Maqui has an antioxidant score (ORAC)* higher than any fruit tested. Maqui berry has the added punch of antioxidants similar to anthocyanins (blueberries), polyphenols, vitamins A & C, iron, potassium and Omega-6.

*AROC Values. 2010.http://oracvalues.com

Antioxidants

Antioxidants are naturally occurring chemicals in foods that counter the negative impact of free radicals in our bodies. Antioxidants keep free radicals from forming in the first place, wipe out current oxidants, and help remove damaged molecules and clean up toxins. The process of oxidation in the human body causes free radicals, which damage cell membranes and other structures. Our bodies are exposed to free radicals naturally through the process of metabolism, and while we can cope with some free radicals, an overload is cause for concern. Factors that increase the presence of free radicals in the body include environmental variables such as pollution, pesticides and radiation, as well as lifestyle factors such as smoking, stress, alcohol and most commonly, poor diet.

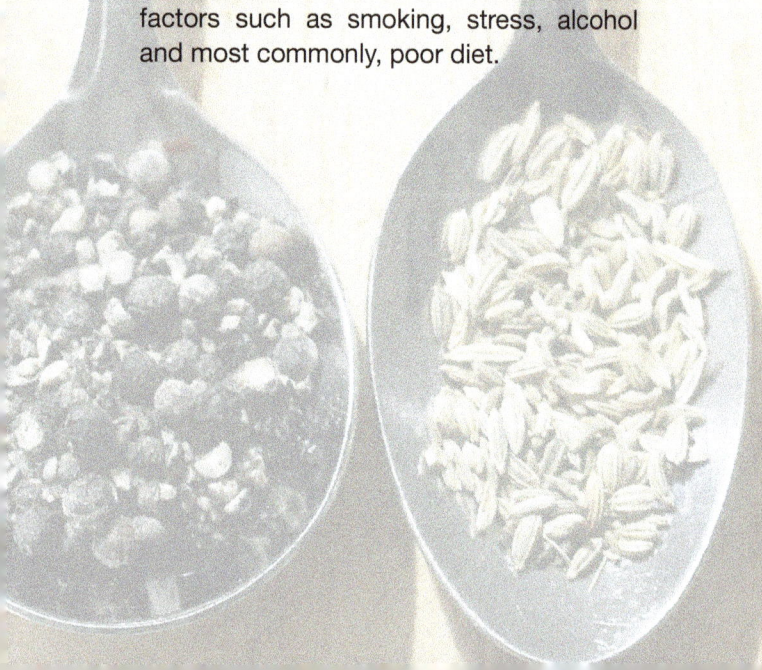

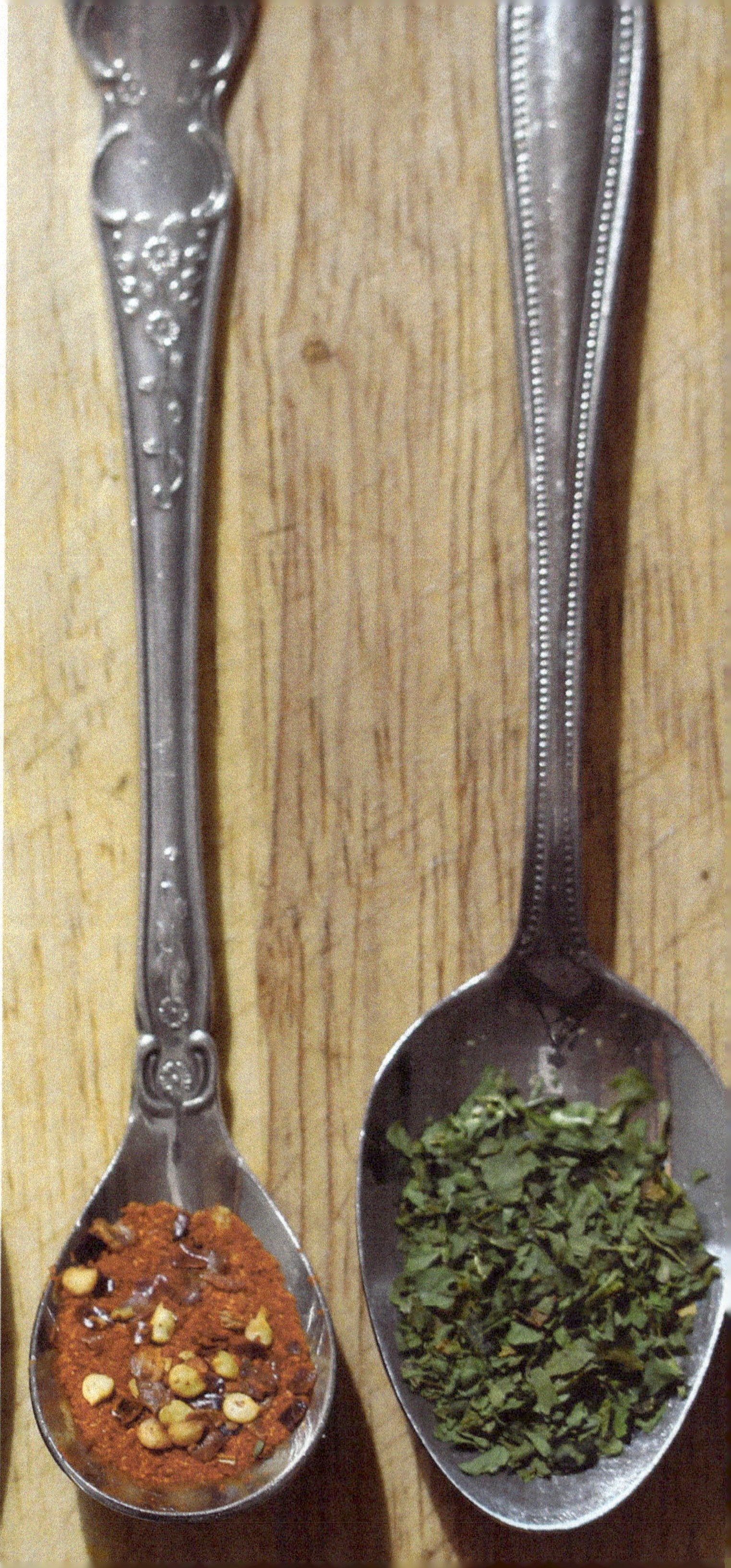

Spices

Adding spices to your food helps to increase the antioxidant levels which in turn helps to keep you both young and healthy. Below is a chart of the top 15 and their ORAC score per only 10 grams.

INGREDIENT Quantity 10 GRAMS	ORAC*
Cloves, ground	26,389
Oregano, dried	15,935
Rosemary, dried	15,025
Thyme, dried	14,307
Cinnamon, ground	11,947
Turmeric, ground	11,551
Vanilla beans, dried	11,127
Nutmeg, ground	6,330
Basil, dried	5,551
Cumin seed	4,579
Ginger, ground	3,549
Pepper, black	3,095
Mustard seed, yellow	2,659
Chilli powder	2,148

*ORAC value is an estimate subject to variance depending on source, growing region, processing procedure, and freshness.

Superfoods

ORAC (Oxygen Radical Absorbance Capacity)

The following scale is used to measure the concentrate levels of antioxidants in foods.

INGREDIENT Quantity 100 GRAMS	ORAC*
Maqui berry powder	612,000
Acai, fruit pulp/skin, powder	102,700
Cacao powder	95,500
Goji berry, raw	25,300
Raspberries, black	19,220
Ginger root, raw	14,840
Chia seed	10,250
Hazelnuts	9,645
Blueberries, wild, raw	9,621
Cranberries, raw	9,090
Almonds	4,454
Strawberries, raw	4,302
Kale	1,770

*ORAC value is an estimate subject to variance depending on source, growing region, processing procedure, and freshness.

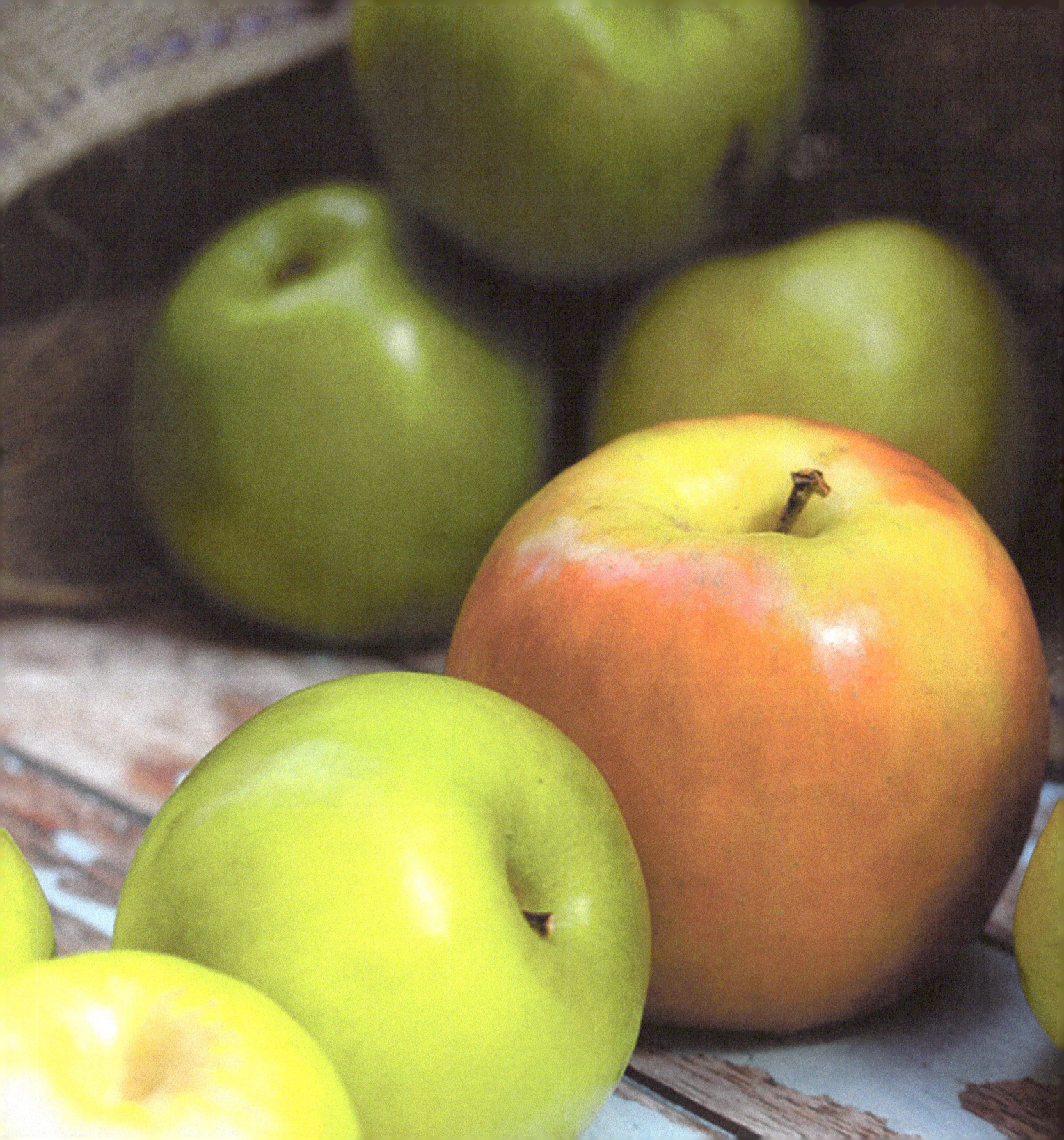

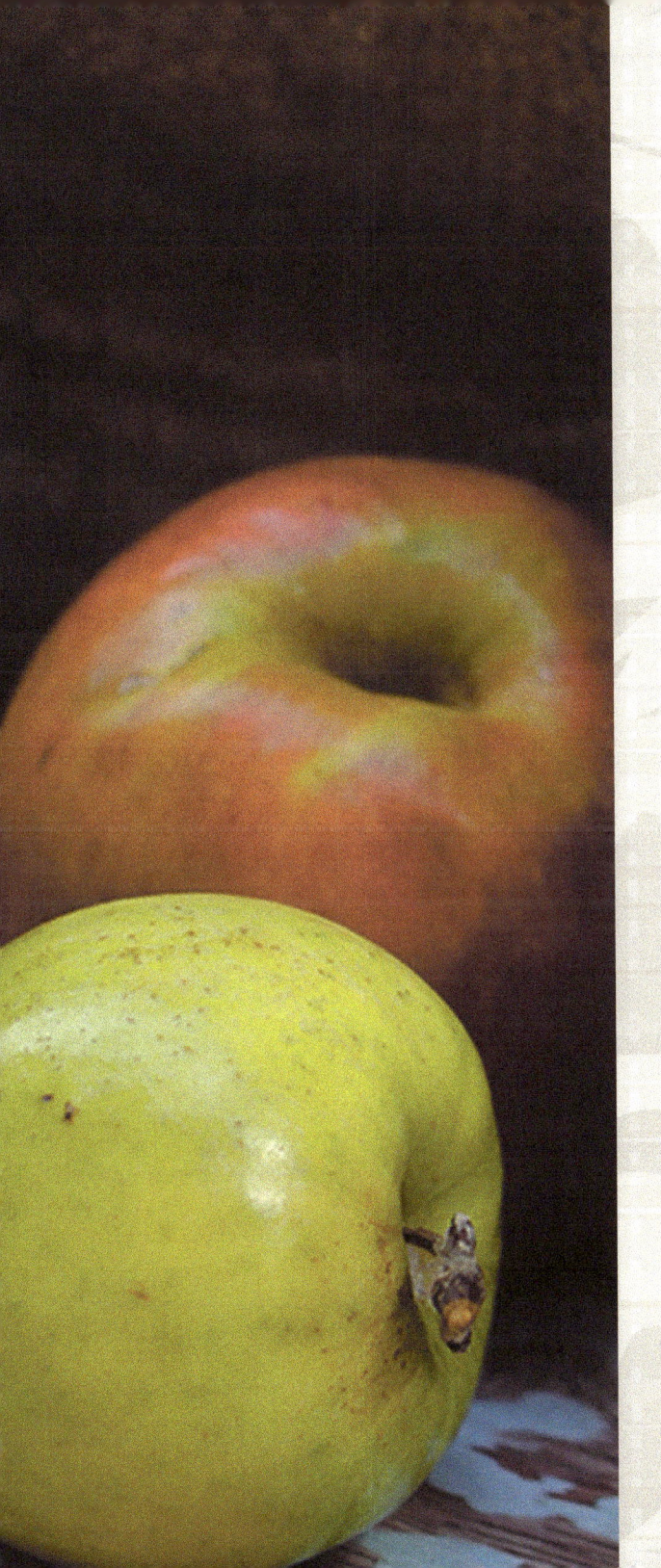

The following symbols are used to indicate which recipes are suitable for different types of diets.

Ⓖ *Grain Free*

Ⓓ *Dairy Free*

Ⓥ *Vegetarian*

(Ve) *Vegan*

(HP) *High Protein*

Ⓢ *Soy Free*

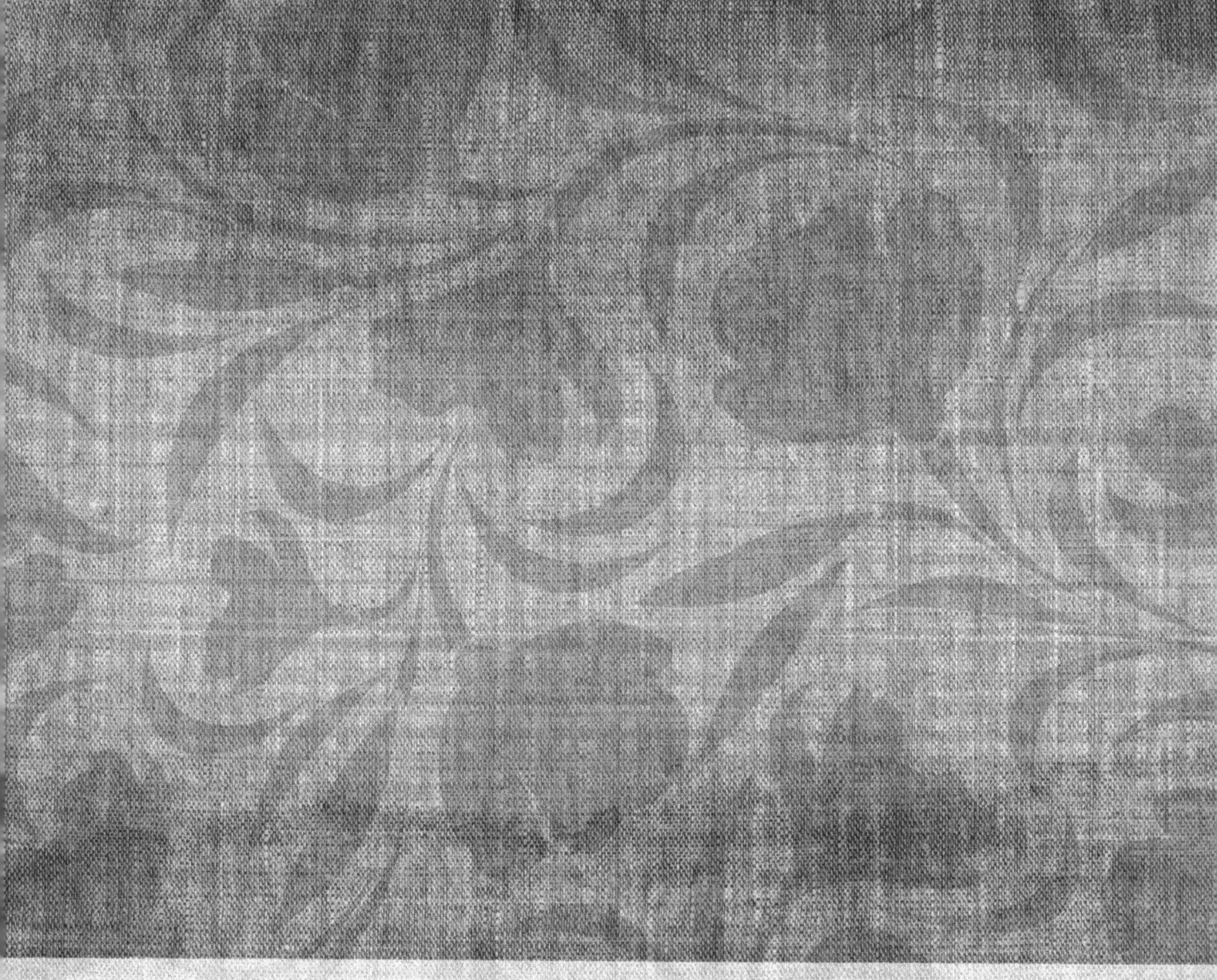

Benefits of blueberries
Blueberries contain the highest antioxidant levels of all fresh fruit: Blueberries, being very rich in anti-oxidants like Anthocyanin, vitamin C, B complex, vitamin E, vitamin A, copper (a very effective immune builder and anti-bacterial), selenium, zinc, iron. Blueberries help to boost your immune system.

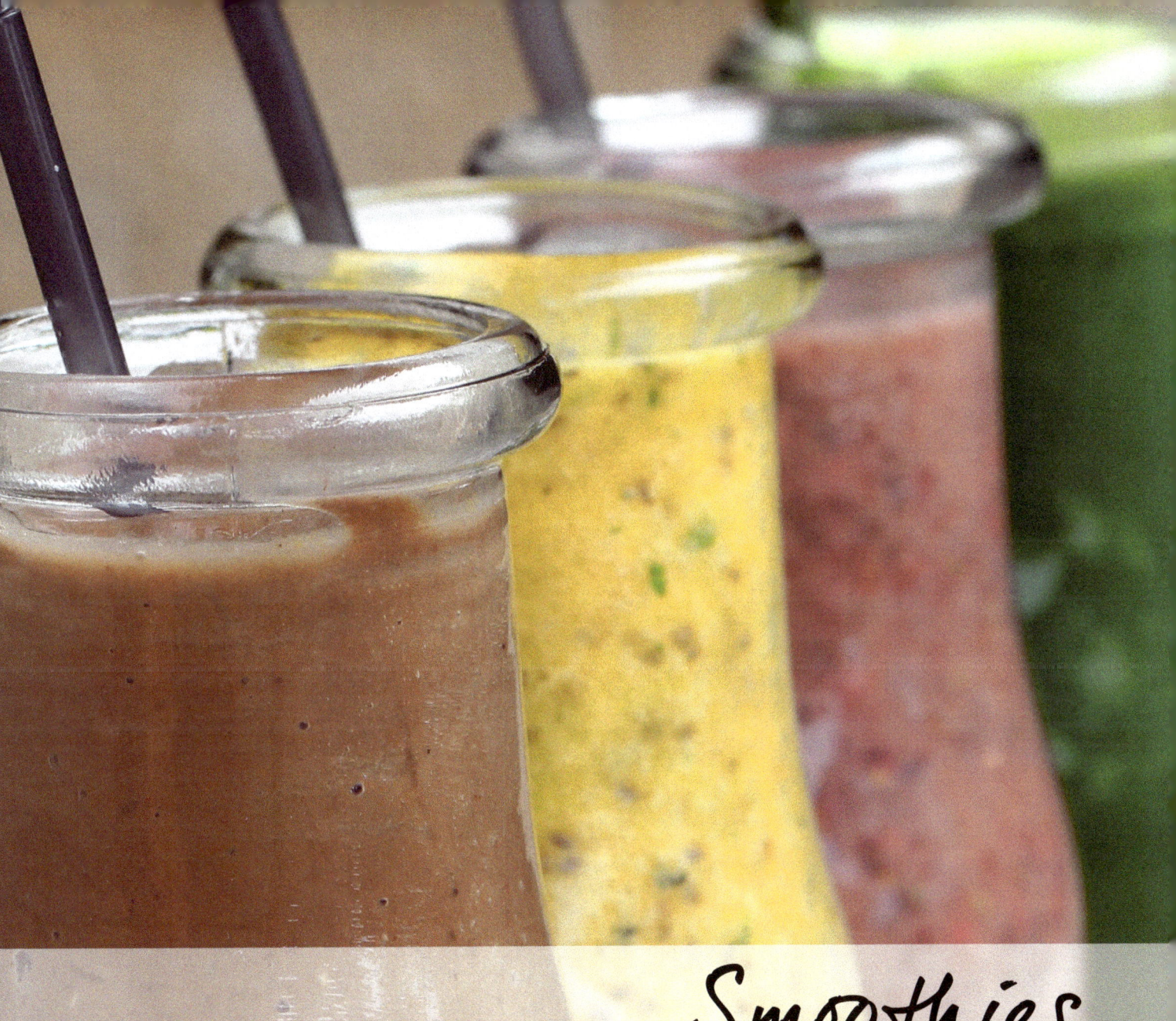

Smoothies & Juices

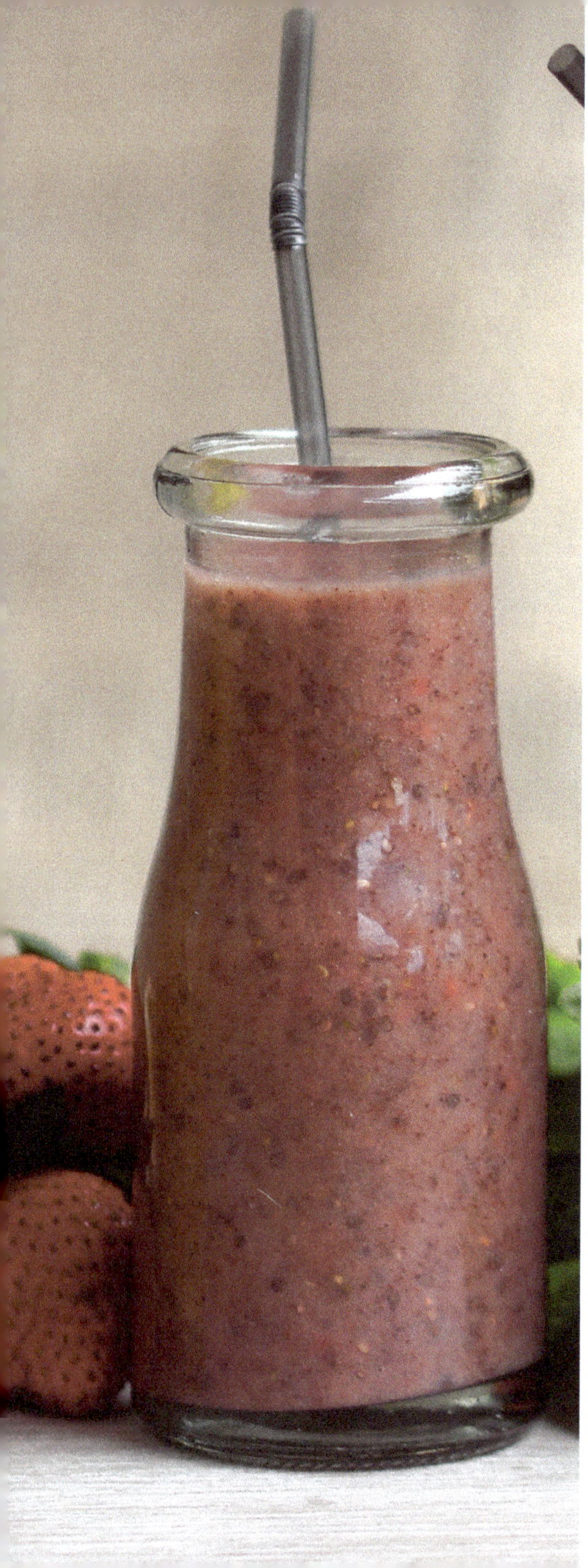

Berry fruit smoothie

Ingredients: 2 serves

1 cup of strawberries
½ cup of mixed blueberries and raspberries (in season)
1 avocado or 1 banana*
1 dessertspoon of chia seeds
2 passion fruit (pulp)
Juice of one lemon
1 teaspoon of organic honey or coconut sugar (optional)
1 teaspoon maqui or acai berry powder
10-15 coconut water ice cubes

Method:
Place ingredients into blender adding ice last on top and blend for 15-20 seconds, adding filtered water as needed and serve.
*banana is higher in the glycemic index

Orange pine smoothie

Ingredients: 2 serves

Juice of one orange
2 teaspoons of goji berries
2 cups of fresh pineapple
4 mint leaves
Juice of ½ lime
5-10 coconut water ice cubes
Two mint leaves
1 dessertspoon of chia seeds (optional)

Method:
Place all ingredients into blender adding ice last on top blend for 15/20 seconds adding filtered water as needed and serve.

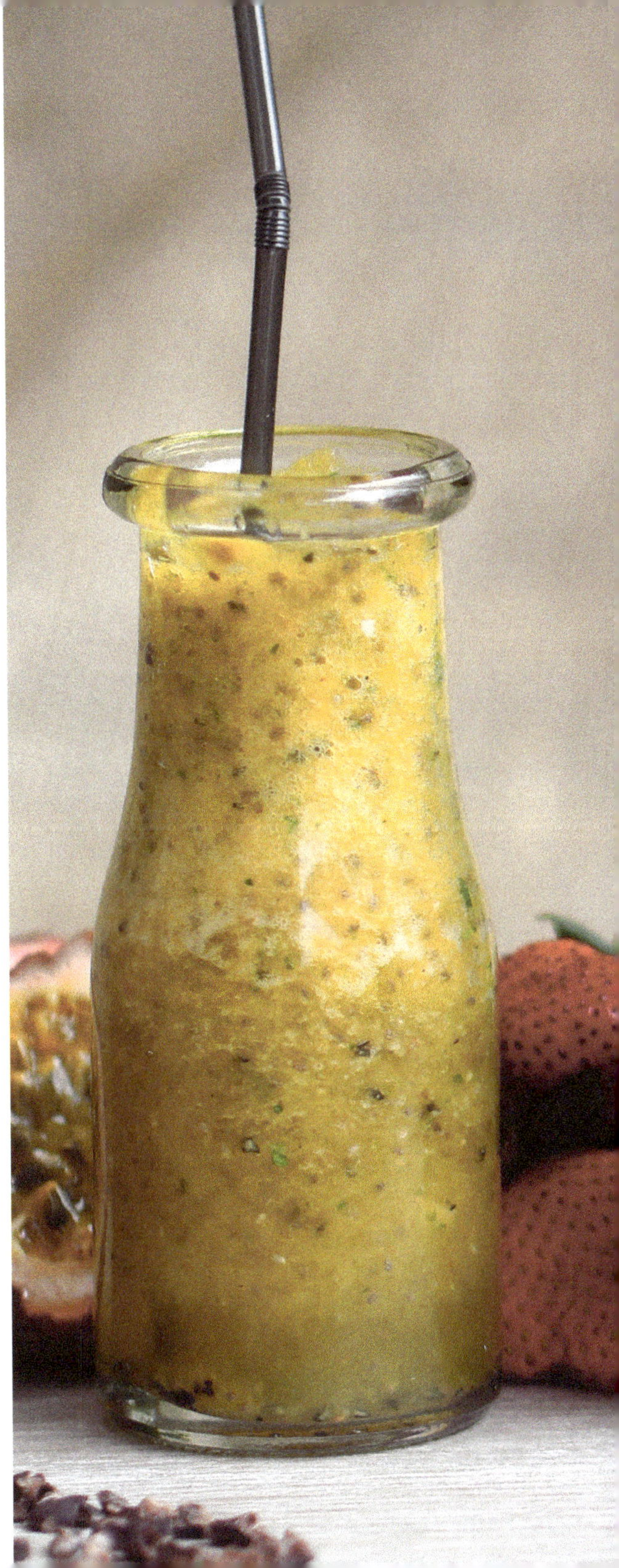

Choc-Berry smoothie

Ingredients: 2 serves

1 cup of strawberries or mixed berries (blue berries/ raspberries)
1 avocado or banana*
1 dessertspoon of organic chia seeds
1 dessertspoon of raw organic cacao powder
2 teaspoons of goji berries
1 cup of coconut water or filtered water
1 teaspoon of maca powder
5-10 ice cubes made from coconut water

Method:
Place all ingredients into blender adding ice last on top blend for 15/20 seconds and serve.
*banana is higher in the glycemic index

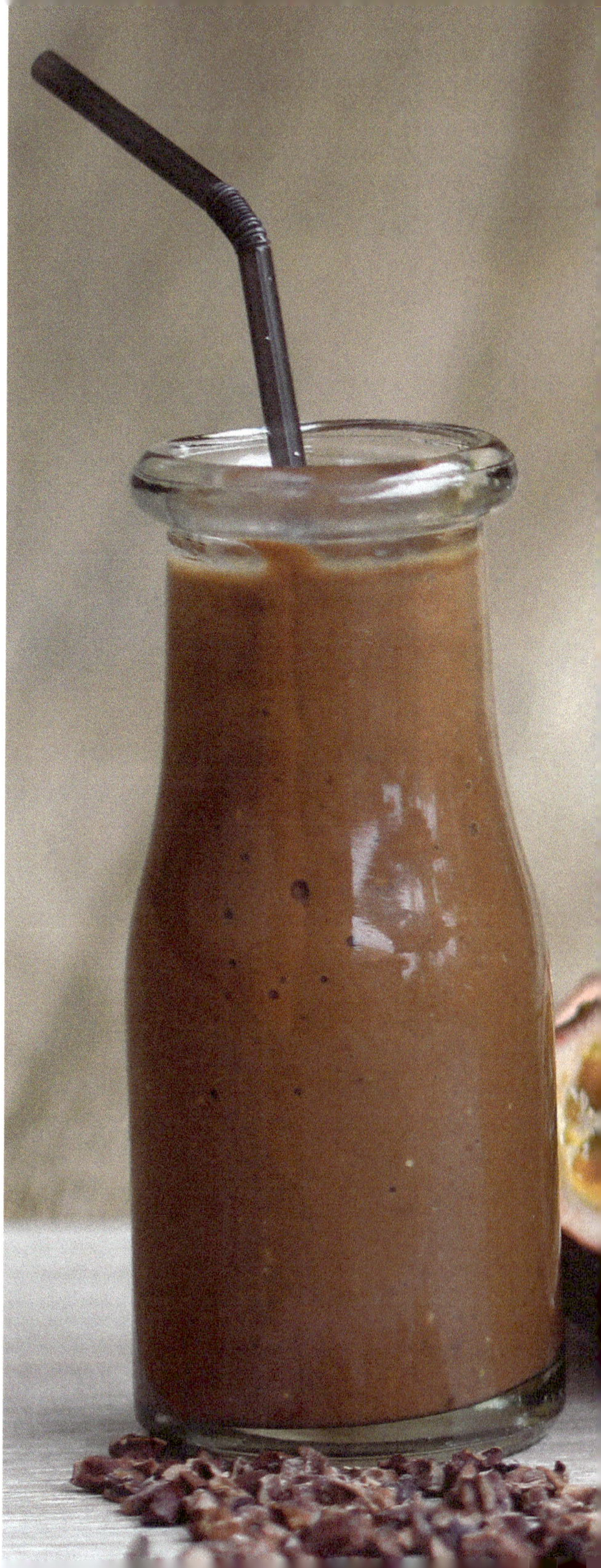

Super green smoothie

Ingredients: 2 serves

1 cup of kale or spinach
1 banana* or avocado
Juice of one lemon
Teaspoon of ginger (optional)
1 dessertspoon of chia seeds
10 mint leaves
10-15 ice cubes made from coconut water

Method:
Place all ingredients into blender adding ice last on top blend for 15/20 seconds adding filtered water as needed and serve.
*banana is higher in the glycemic index

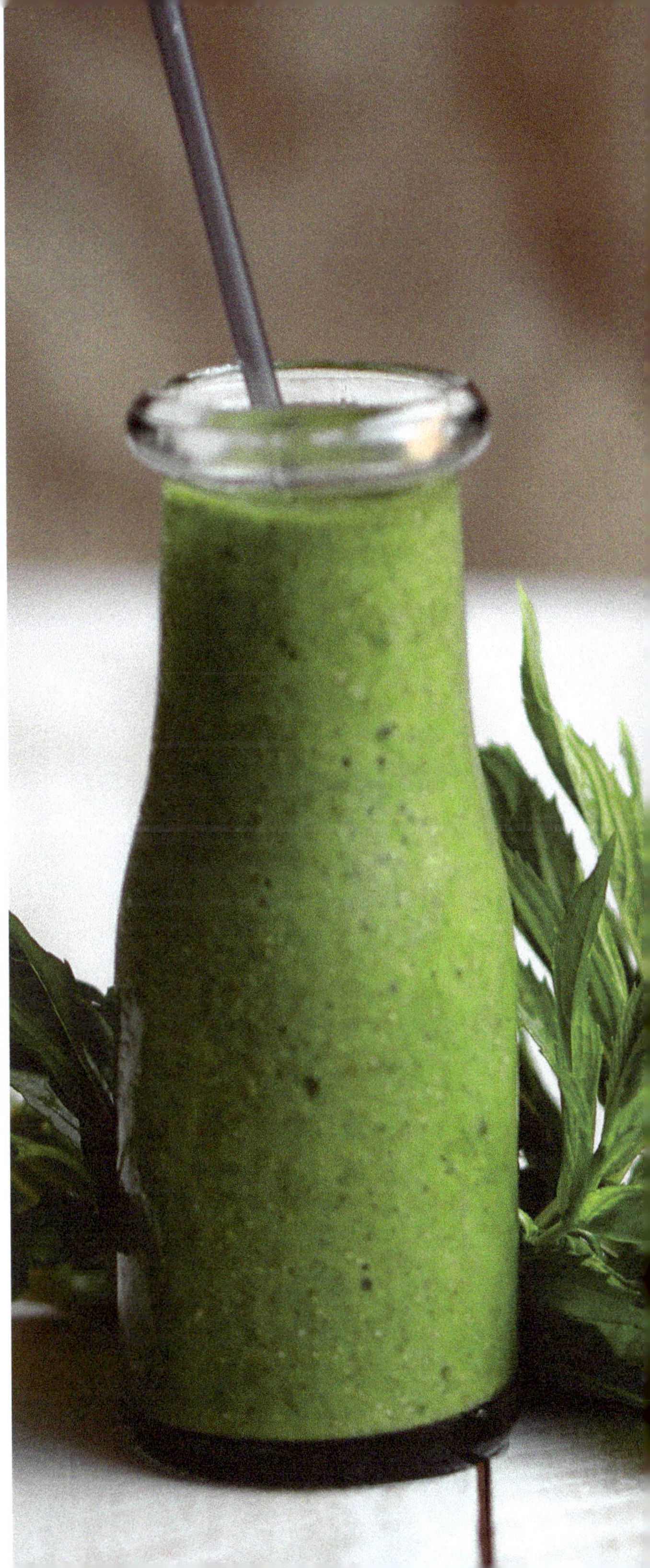

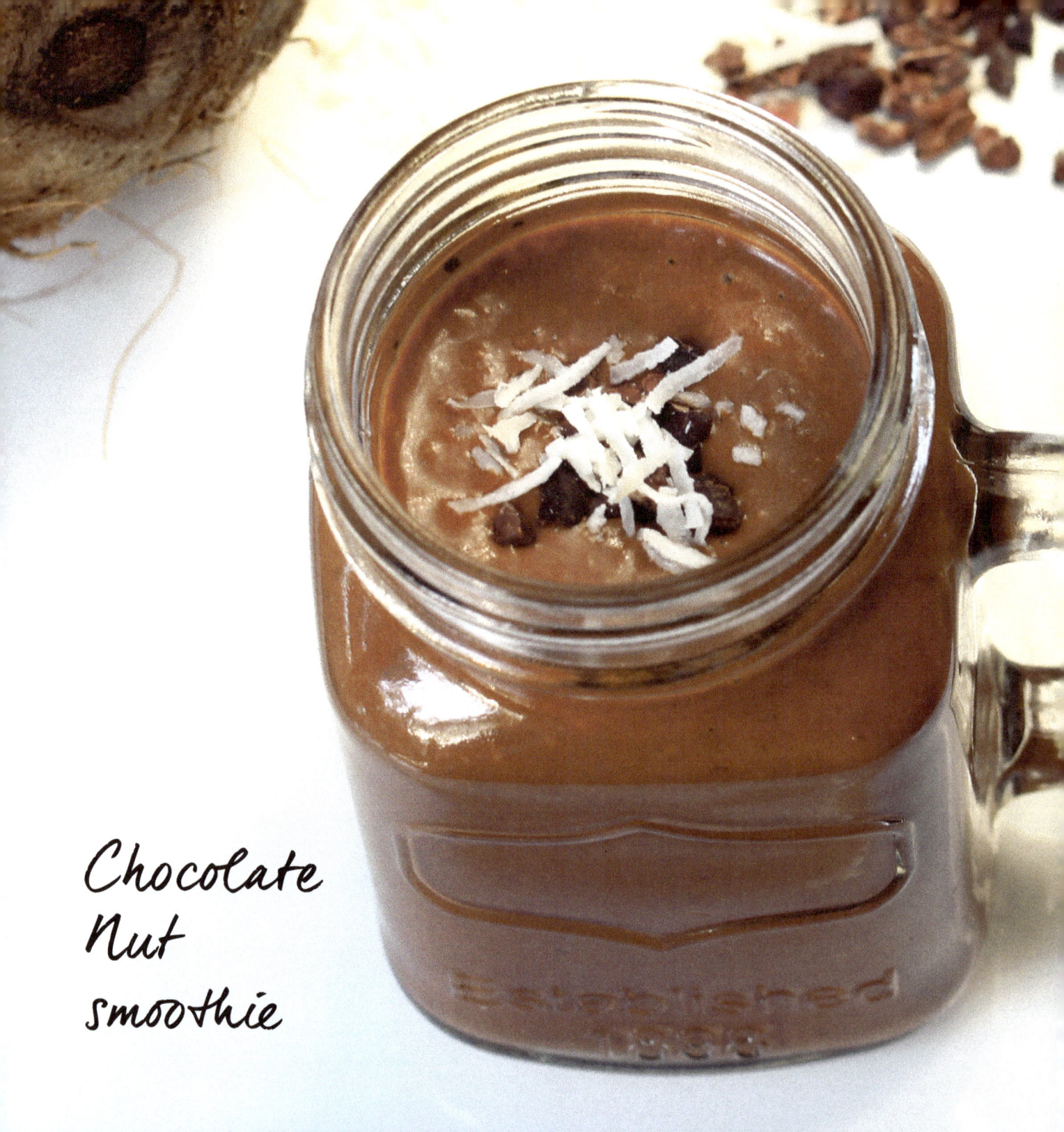

Chocolate Nut smoothie

Chocolate nut smoothie

Ingredients: 2 serves

1 banana* or avocado
½ cup of mixed nuts
1 dessertspoon of chia seeds
1 desertsoon of organic cacao powder
1 tablespoon of protein powder (optional)
1 teaspoon of nut butter (macadamia or almond) optional
1 teaspoon of organic honey or coconut sugar (vegan)
10 ice cubes made from coconut water and half cup of water or coconut water

Method:
Place all ingredients into blender adding ice last on top blend for 15/20 seconds and serve.
*banana is higher in the glycemic index

Pear & cinnamon chia smoothie

Ingredients: 2 serves

2 soft pears
1 teaspoon of ground cinnamon
1 teaspoon of ground vanilla bean (or vanilla extract)
1 cup of fresh apple juice
1 dessertspoon of chia seeds
1 teaspoon of raw honey (optional) or coconut sugar (vegan)
4-6 coconut ice cubes

Method:
Place all ingredients into blender adding ice last on top. Blend for 15/20 seconds and serve.

Banana coconut smoothie

Ingredients: 1-2 serves

1 banana
1 cup of coconut milk
1 dessertspoon of shredded coconut
1 tablespoon of Raw organic cacao powder
1 teaspoon of maca powder
4-6 ice cubes made from coconut water

Method:
Place ingredients into blender ice cubes on top and blend for 10-20 seconds until creamy texture.

Breakfast detox juice

Ingredients: 2 serves

2 sticks of celery
½ small beetroot
1 whole lemon
1 medium carrot
1 apple (optional)
1 teaspoon size of raw ginger
1 teaspoon size of raw turmeric
or ½ teaspoon of powder
1 dessertspoon chia seeds
1 teaspoon maca powder
2 dessertspoons of pulp extracted from juicer (for fibre)
1 teaspoon of alkalizing greens powder (optional)
Sprinkle of ground chilli (optional)

Method:
Place all vegetables through juicer, pour juice into glass and add chia seeds, maca powder, chilli, and greens powders, also add two dessertspoons of pulp extracted from vegetables to glass and mix well. This juice is a great tangy energy boost to start the day. Add or adjust quantities to suit your palate.

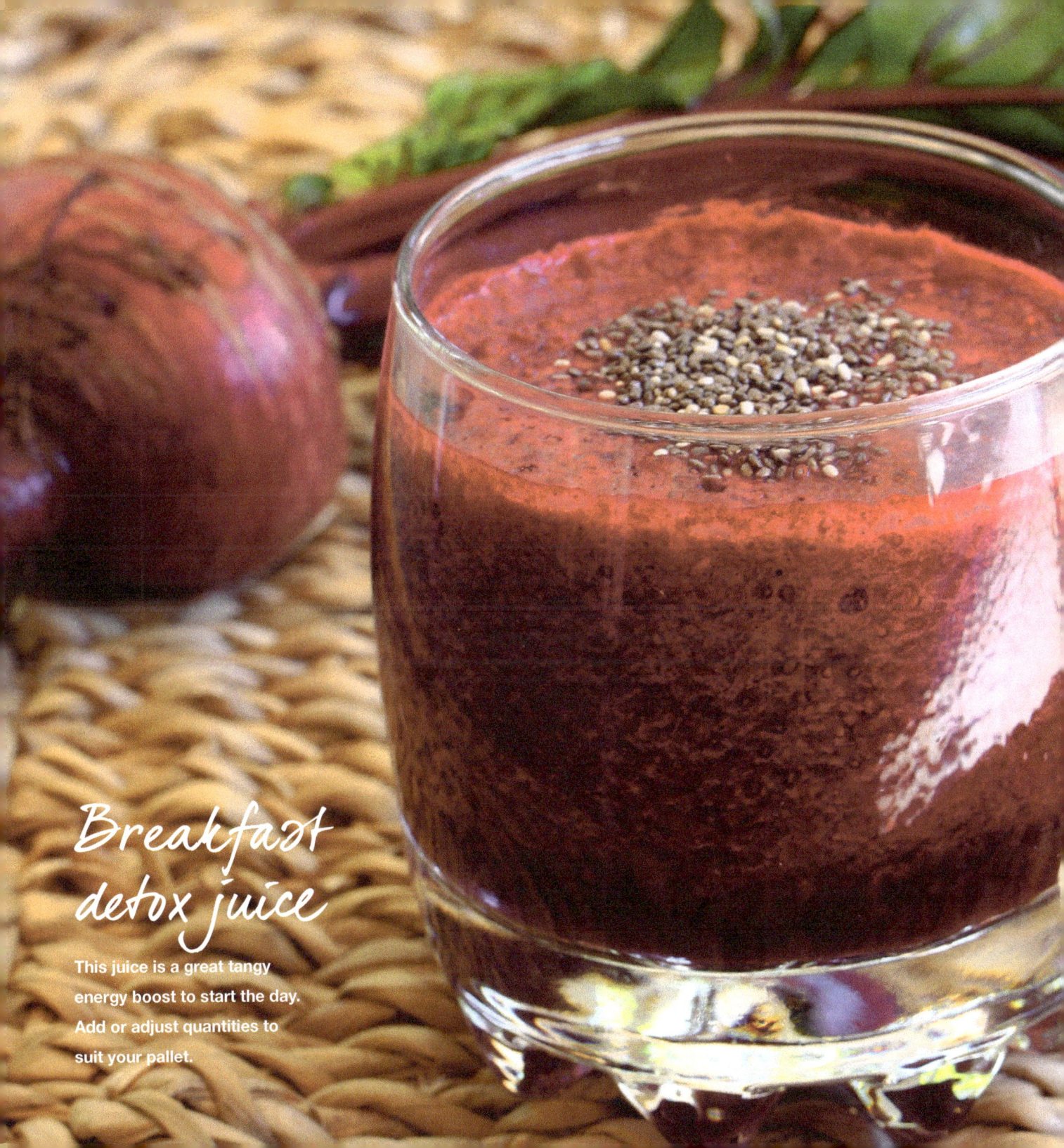

Breakfast detox juice

This juice is a great tangy energy boost to start the day. Add or adjust quantities to suit your pallet.

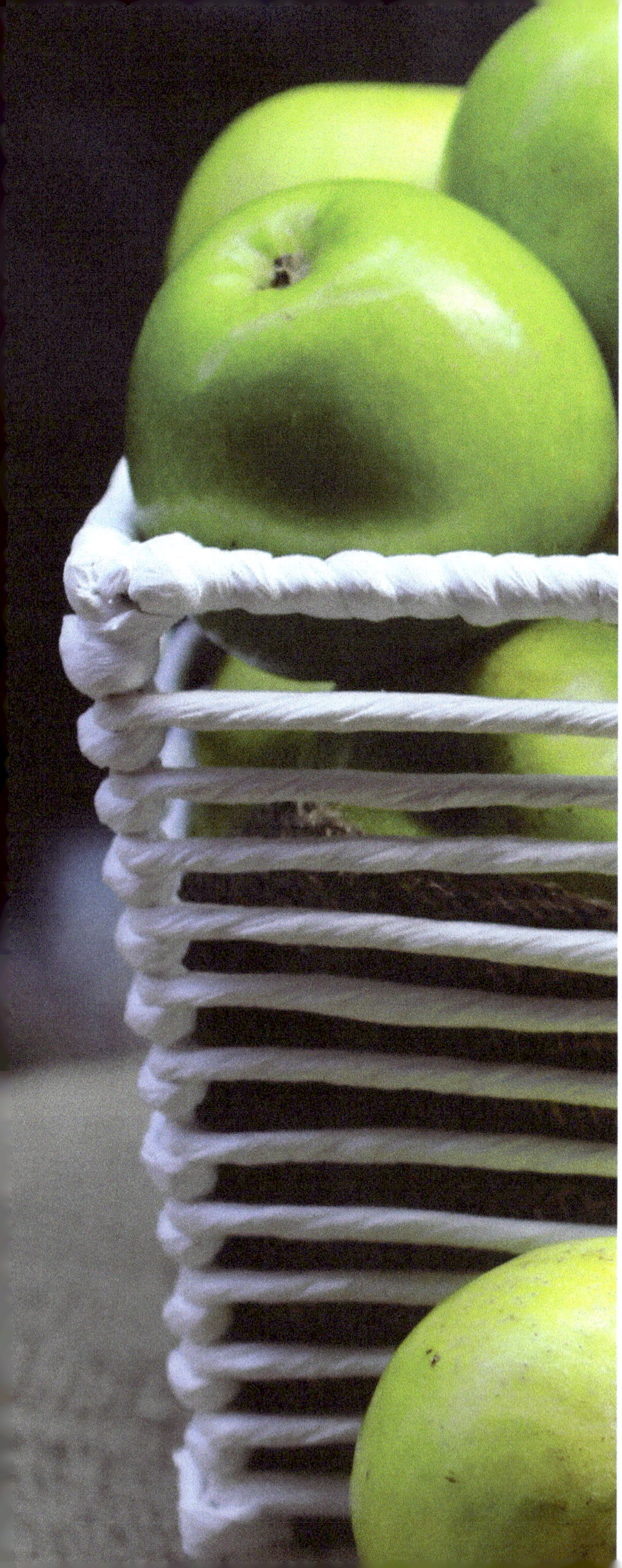

Apple celery carrot juice

Ingredients: 1 serve

1 apple
1 medium carrot
2 sticks of celery
1 dessertspoon of chia seeds
1 teaspoon of apple cider vinegar
1 teaspoon of maca powder

Method:
Place fruit and vegetables through juicer
Add in apple cider vinegar and maca powder and chia seeds.
Drink straight away to gain the maximum benefit from the nutrients.

Green tea, mint smoothie

Ingredients: 2 Serves

2 teaspoons of green tea leaves
2 cups baby spinach leaves or Kale
4 mint leaves
Juice of 1 a lemon
¼ cup of cucumber
1 dessertspoon of chia seeds
4-6 ice cubes

Method:
Place all ingredients into blender adding ice last on top blend for 15/20 seconds and serve.

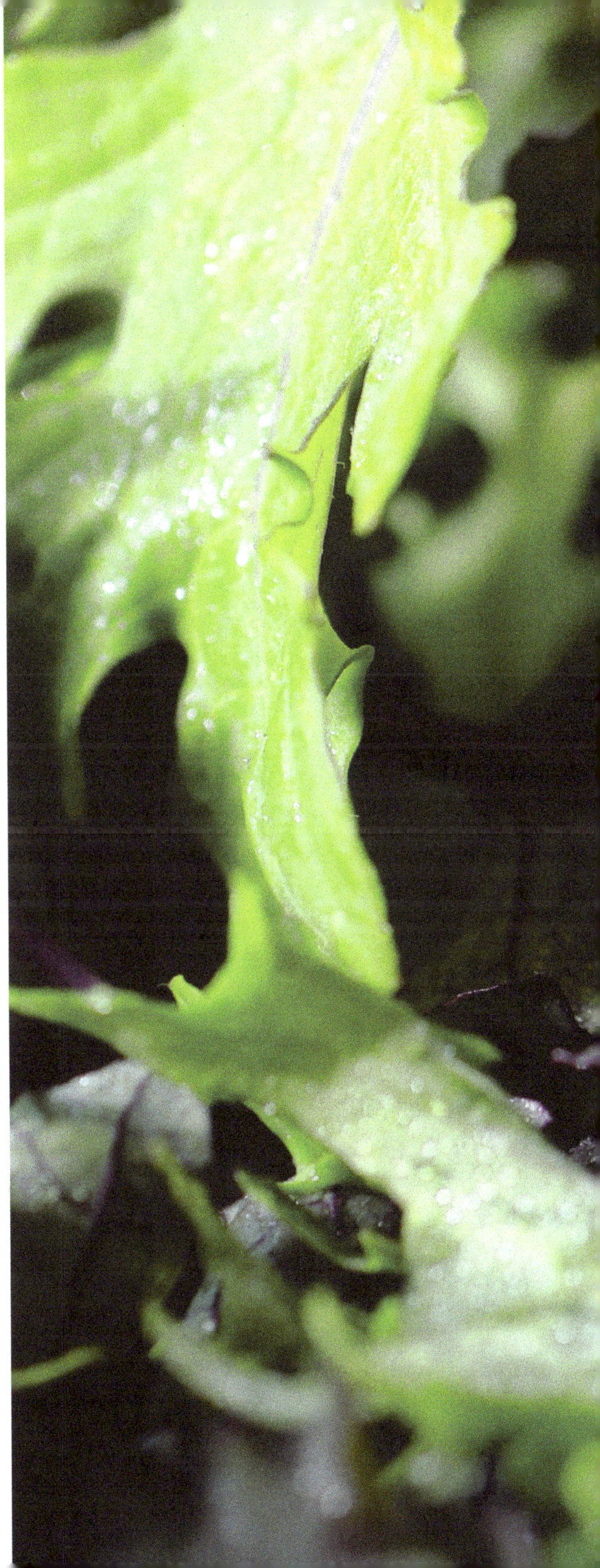

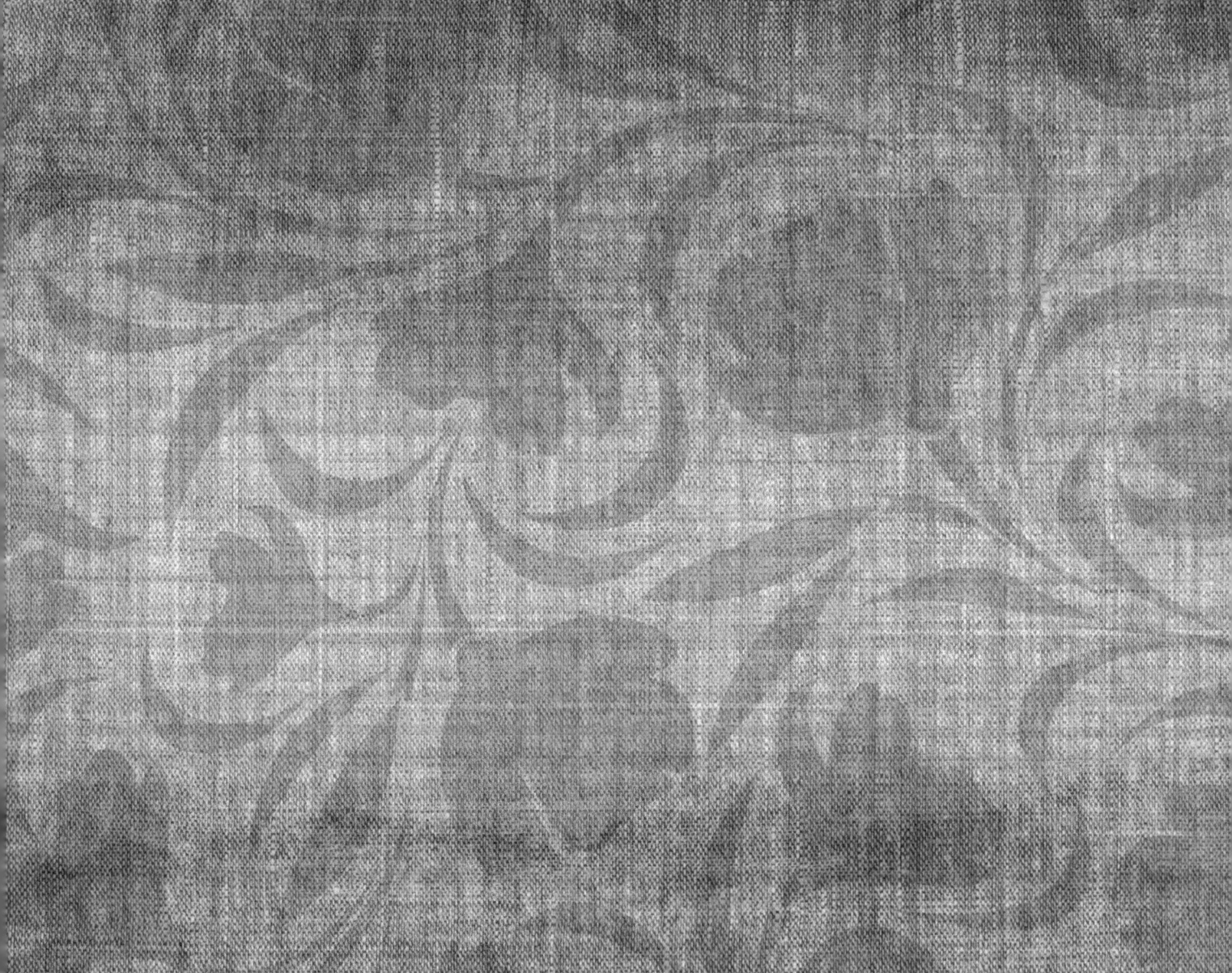

The Importance of water

*"Without water nothing lives." Water is our main source of energy, creating electrical and magnetic energy inside every cell of the body. Water prevents DNA damage, and greatly increases the efficiency of the immune system in the bone marrow. Water energizes food and food particles are then able to supply the body with this energy during digestion. Water helps reduce the risk of heart attacks and stroke. Water is the main lubricant in the joint spaces and helps prevent arthritis and back pain. These are just some of the reasons why your body needs water every day.

*Batmanghlidj,F MD. And Phillip Day. The Essential Guide to Water and Salt. Kent, Great Britain; Credence Publications, 2008

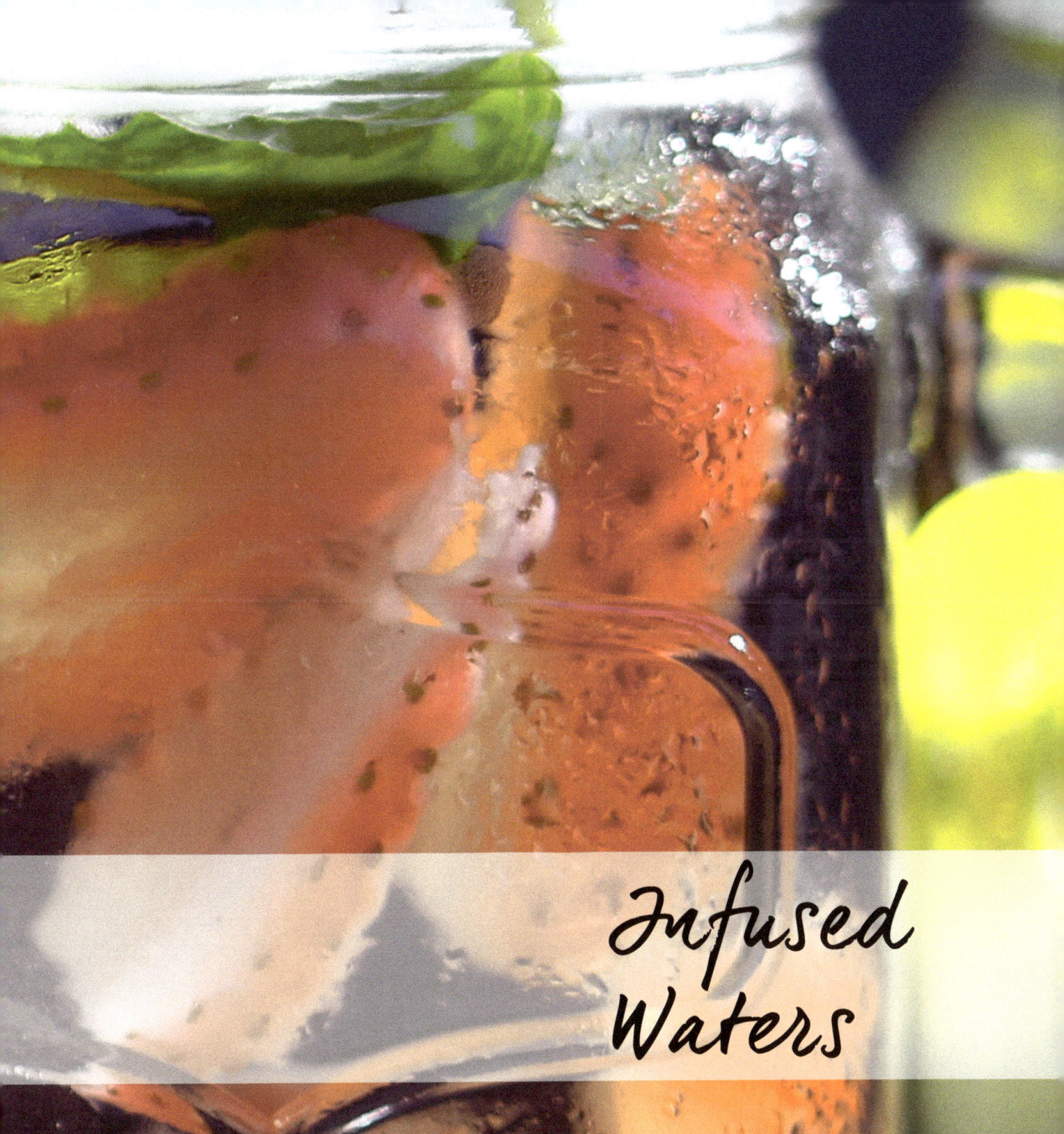

Infused Waters

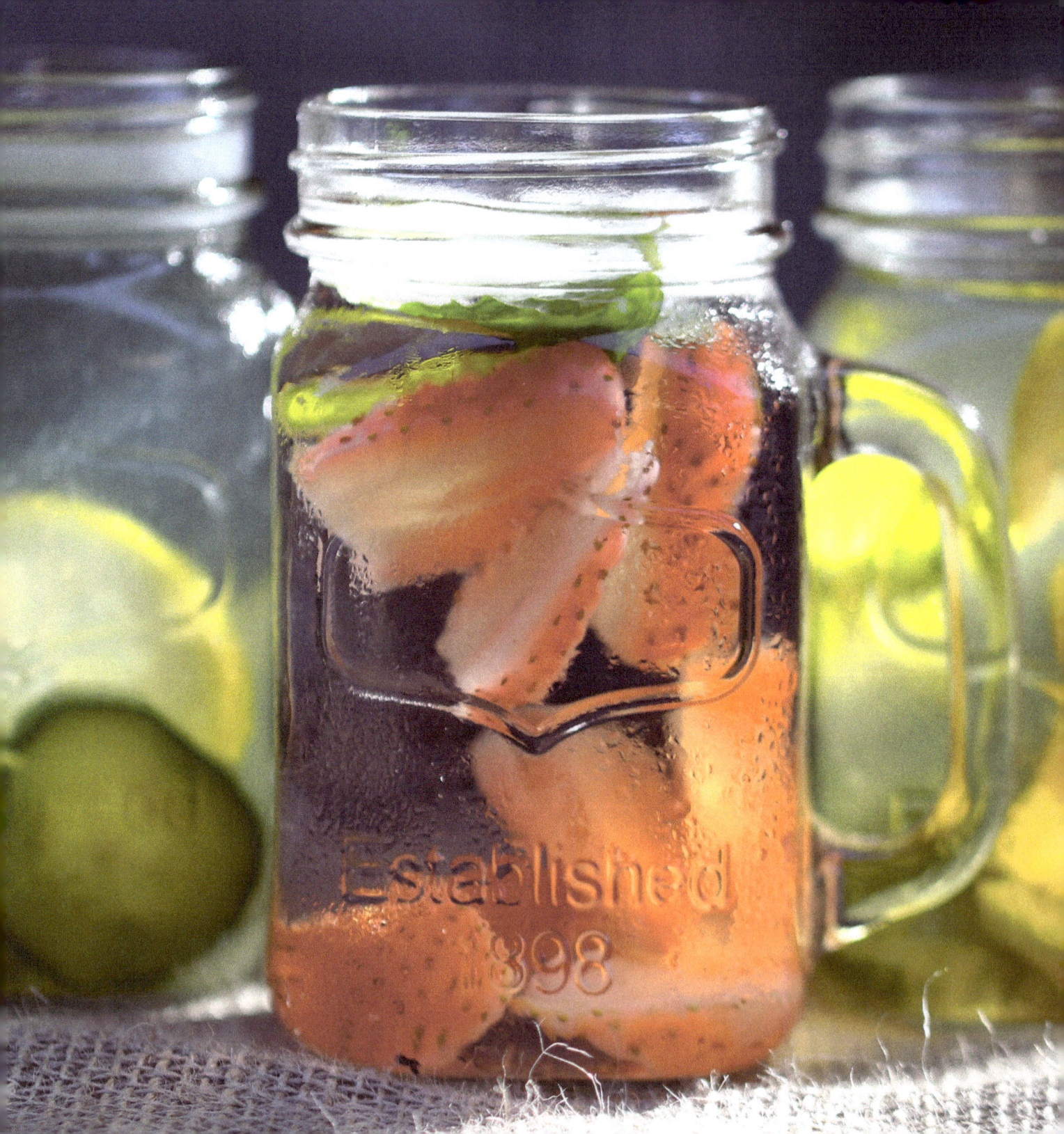

Berry water

Ingredients:

2 strawberries sliced in half
1 mint leaf
1 cup of coconut water or filtered water
Coconut water
ice cubes to chill

Method:
Place ingredients together in glass bottle in store in fridge for 1-2 hours.
A light refreshing drink.

Lemon cucumber water

Ingredients:

Juice of half one lemon
2 slices of lemon
1 slice of cucumber
1 cup of coconut water or filtered water.
Coconut water / ice cubes to chill

Method:
Place ingredients together in glass bottle in store in fridge for 1-2 hours
A light refreshing drink.

Green tea with lemon & mint water

Ingredients:

1 cup of green tea
1 mint leaf
2 slices of lemon or lime

Method:
Make up green tea and let cool, then add slice of lemon or lime and one mint leaf and chill in fridge in a glass jar for 1-2 hours. This is a very refreshing light drink on a hot day.

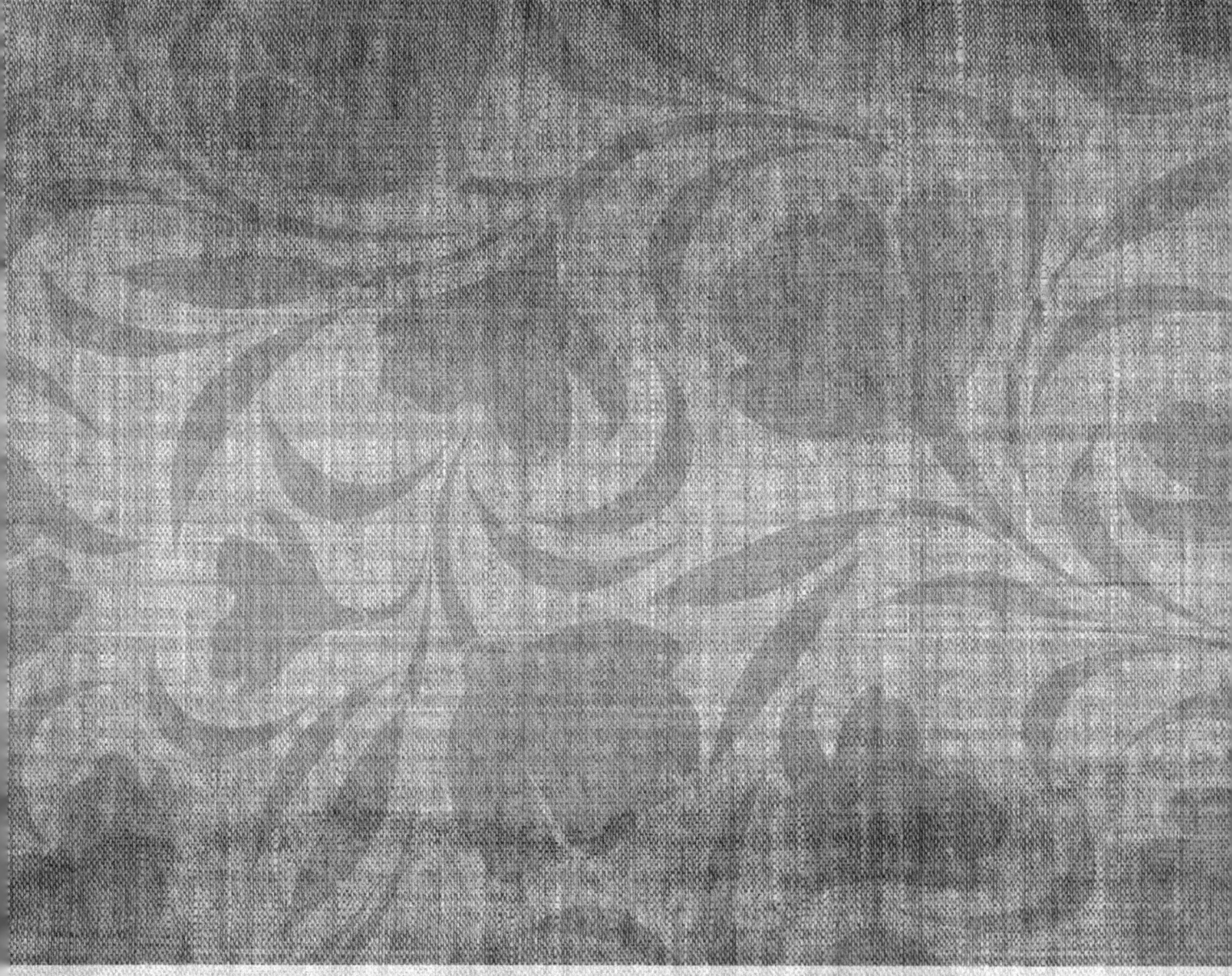

Benefits of almonds & hazelnuts

Almonds are high in vitamins, minerals, and dietary fibre. Almonds contain a high quality protein and high levels of healthy unsaturated fatty acids for a healthy heart.

Hazelnuts similar to the almond are also rich in vitamins and minerals. Hazelnuts contain unsaturated fatty acids for a healthy heart.

Almonds and hazelnuts contain magnesium for bone and joint health, as well as high levels of vitamin E for healthy Skin. The B vitamins help to lessen stress, anxiety and depression.

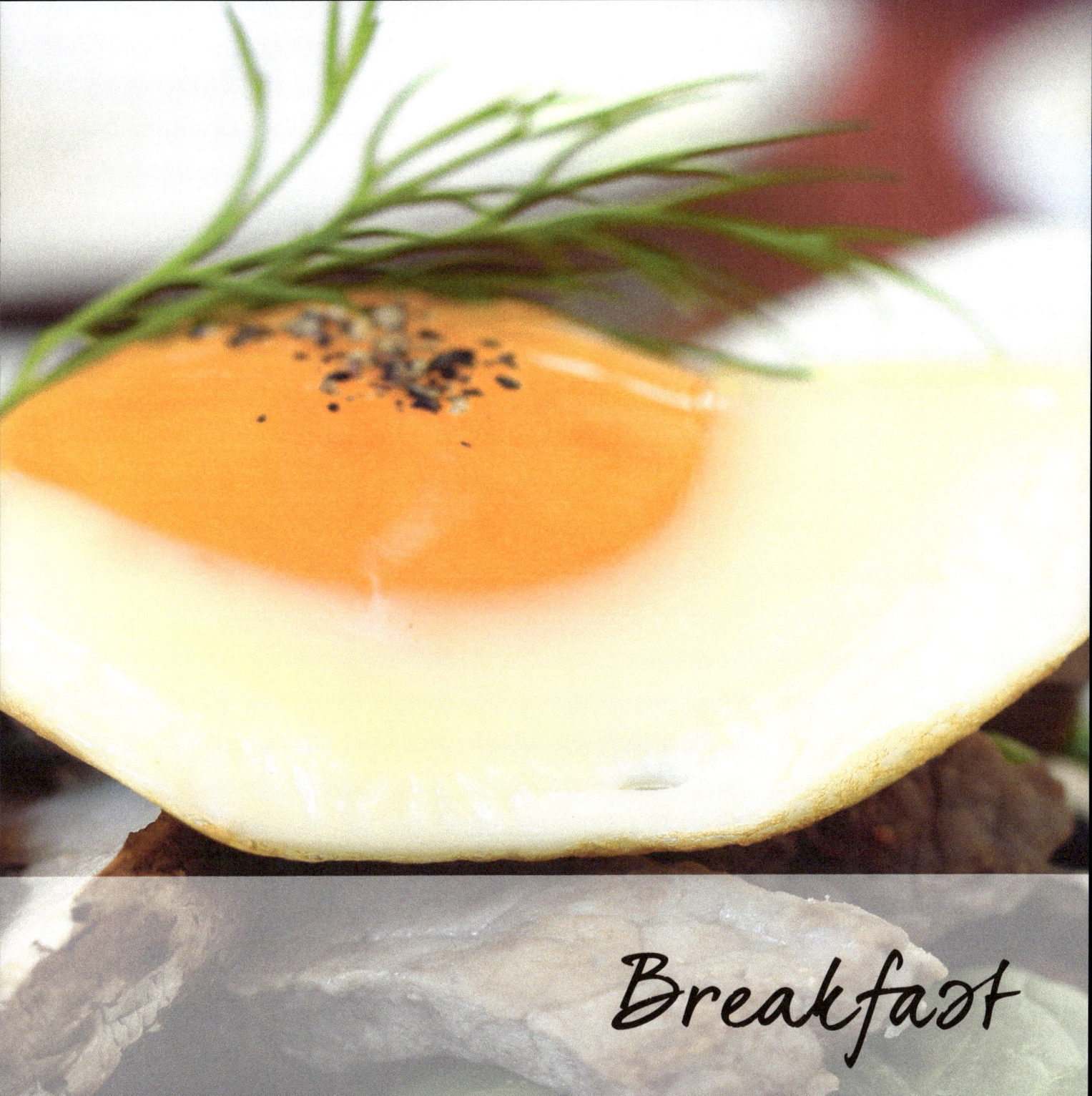

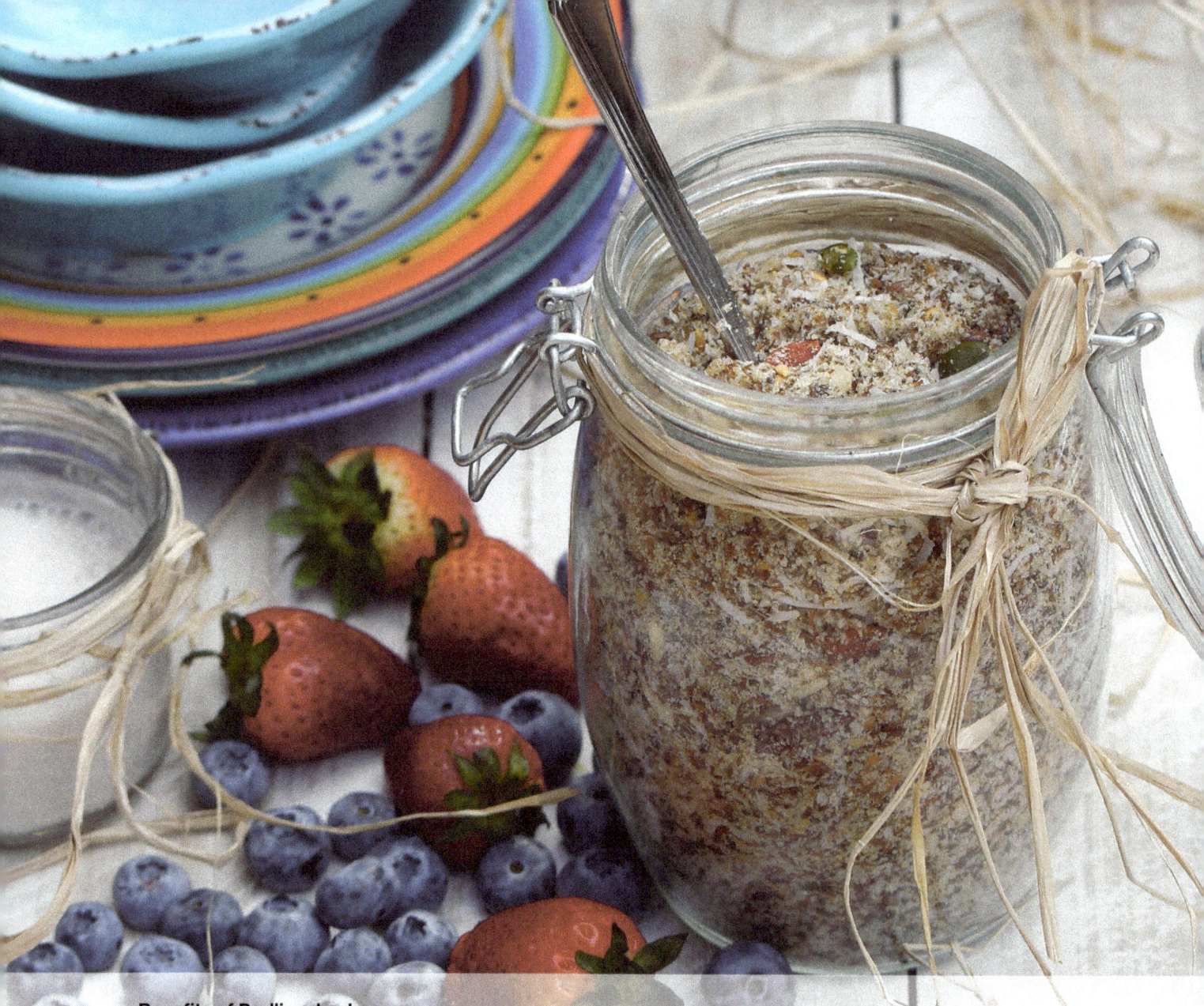

Benefits of Psyllium husks

Psyllium is a herb used in weight control and for general intestinal health. It contains a spongy fibre that reduces appetite, improves digestion and cleanses the system, making it an excellent choice for a healthy diet. Psyllium husk is high in fibre. This is great in assisting in obtaining a healthy gut. Research suggests* that dietary fibre contains a unique blend of bioactive components including resistant starches, vitamins, minerals, phytochemicals and antioxidants, having a positive effect on metabolism.

*James M. Lattimer and Mark D. Haub Review effects of dietary fibre and its components on metabolic health Nutrients 2010

Grain free muesli

Ingredients:

½ cup of almond meal

½ cup hazelnut meal

¼ cup sunflower seeds

¼ cup sesame seeds

¼ cup of pepitas (pumpkin seeds)

¼ cup chia seeds

¼ cup brazil nuts

½ cup of coconut slithers

½ cup psyllium husks

½ cup of Flax seed meal

¼ cup goji Berries

¼ cup linseeds

5 tablespoons of coconut oil

Teaspoon of organic vanilla extract if desired (optional)

Optional 1/4 cup sultanas or dates chopped to sweeten (optional)

Method:

Place Brazil nuts, pumpkin seeds in blender for 5 seconds and mix in with all other ingredients together. Then add the coconut oil stirring it in until small clusters form. Place in airtight container in the fridge.
For toasted muesli place mixture on a tray and put into an oven at 55 degrees for 2-4 hours then turn off oven and leave inside for another two hours. When cooled down place in airtight container in the fridge. Serve with almond or coconut milk and fresh fruit in season.

Note: Coconut oil is a solid when room temperature is less than 18 degrees Celsius, place jar in a small bowl of hot water for a couple of minutes to liquefy.

High protein salmon omelet

Ingredients: 1-2 serves

3-4 eggs

2 dessertspoons of water (filtered preferred)

1 tablespoon of chopped parsley

1 spring onion sliced

¼ cup of diced red capsicum

100 grams of sliced smoked salmon

6-8 baby spinach leaves

2 sliced mushrooms (optional)

Pink mineral salt & pepper to taste

Sprinkle of chilli (optional)

2 dessertspoons of sauerkraut

4-5 Cherry tomatoes

¼ cup of diced cucumber

Juice of half a lemon

Method:

Place eggs into a small bowl and add water pepper, salt wick well. Prepare diced filling ingredients and set aside. Place pan on medium low heat add coconut oil. Then add salmon and lightly cook for a few minutes. Next add egg mixture to pan, followed by capsicum, onion, and parsley. Once egg mixture has cooked, add baby spinach leaves and fold in half and serve on top of a bed of sauerkraut (2 dessertspoons) and side serve of baby cherry tomatoes or diced tomatoes and cucumber with a squeeze of lemon juice.

Grain free pancakes

Ingredients: 1-2 serves

½ cup of coconut flour

½ cup of organic blanched almond meal

4 eggs

1 teaspoon of bi-carb soda

2 cups of almond milk

1 teaspoon of organic vanilla extract (optional)

½ teaspoon of ground cinnamon (optional)

2 tablespoons of chia seeds

1 cup of blueberries (optional)

Method:

Place dry ingredients into glass mixing bowl, add eggs slowly using hand mixer or whisker, and then slowly add milk while mixing. Mix until smooth consistency leave to stand for 5 minutes. Heat a pan to medium heat place a teaspoon of coconut oil to melt then place a spoonful of mixture into pan, once air bubbles appear on top flip pancake and cook until golden brown.

Serve with organic honey/coconut sugar and lemon juice or I cup of berries blended into sauce. Another option is sliced banana or orange segments.

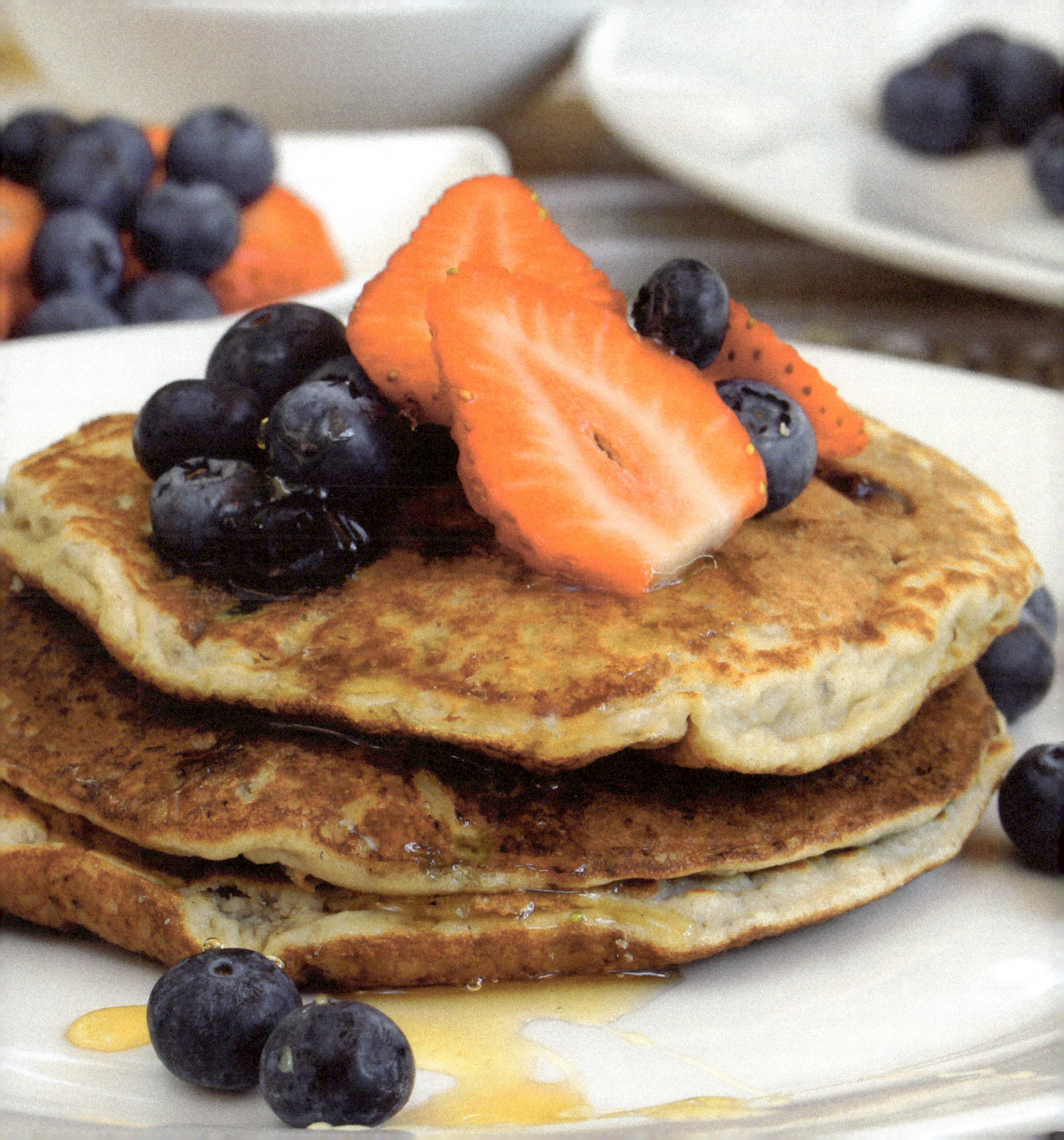

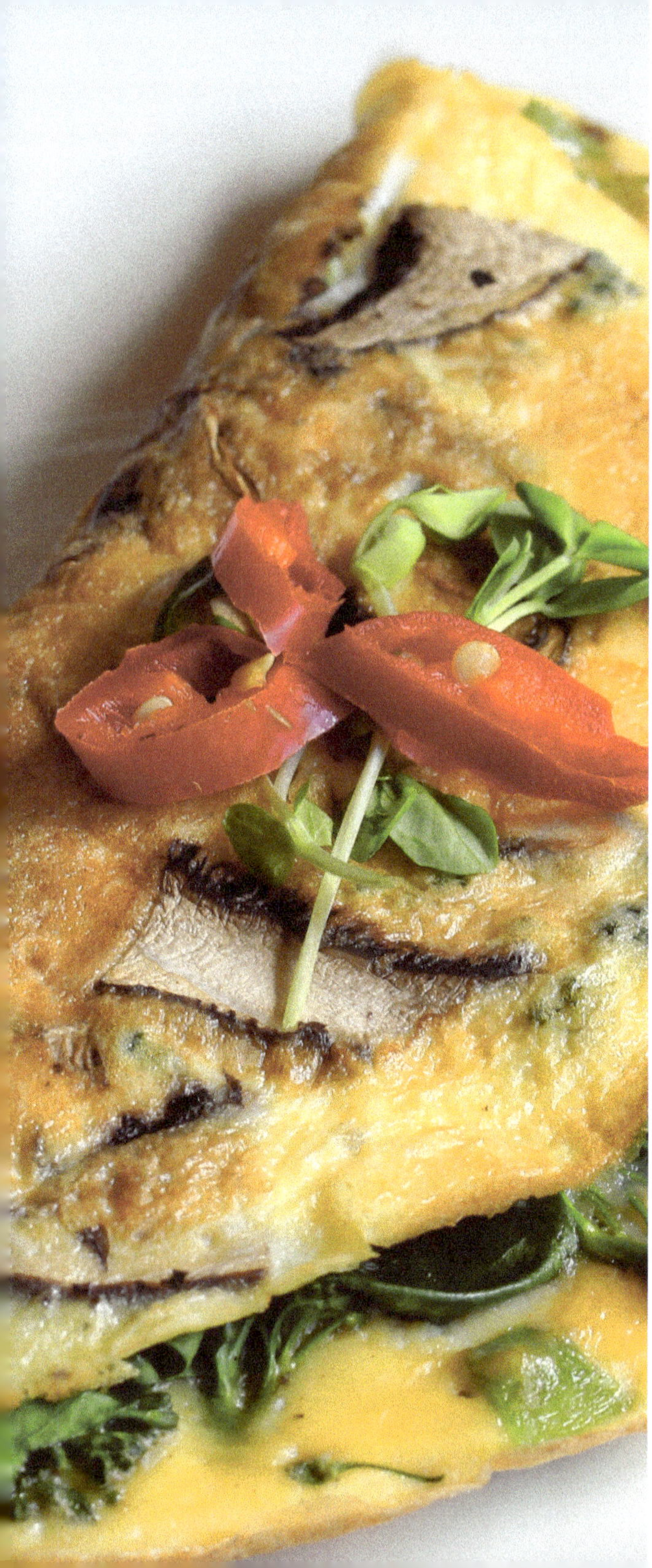

Breakfast omelet

Ingredients: 2 serves
4 eggs
2 tablespoons water (filtered preferred)
½ cup of diced red & green capsicum
1-2 mushrooms sliced
¼ cup of finely chopped broccoli
8-10 sliced baby spinach leaves
½ of a tomato diced (optional)
Pinch of pink mineral salt and cracked pepper to taste
Sprinkle of chilli and chia seeds (optional)
1 teaspoon of coconut oil

Method:
Place eggs into a small bowl and add water pepper, salt and chilli and whisk well. Prepare diced filling ingredients and set aside. Place pan on heat add coconut oil. Then add egg mixture to pan, followed by diced capsicum, onion, broccoli, mushrooms and tomato. Once egg mixture has cooked add spinach leaves and fold in half and serve.

High Protein option add cooked chicken for an even heartier start to your day. This can even be an evening meal option as well.

Beef strips with egg & spinach

Ingredients: 1 serve (double quantities for 2 serves)

1-2 eggs
100g beef topside strips
1 tomato
2 small mushrooms diced
½ cup baby spinach leaves
¼ of a grated carrot
¼ of a small grated beetroot
Pinch of pink mineral salt and cracked pepper to taste

Method:

Place beef strips into heated pan on medium heat, and then add mushroom, tomato. After a couple of minutes add the eggs and cook until whites are set. Then place Beef on top of baby spinach leaves followed by eggs, tomatoes, mushrooms,

Optional fresh grated carrot and grated beetroot. Sprinkle with chilli, pinch of pink mineral salt and cracked pepper to taste

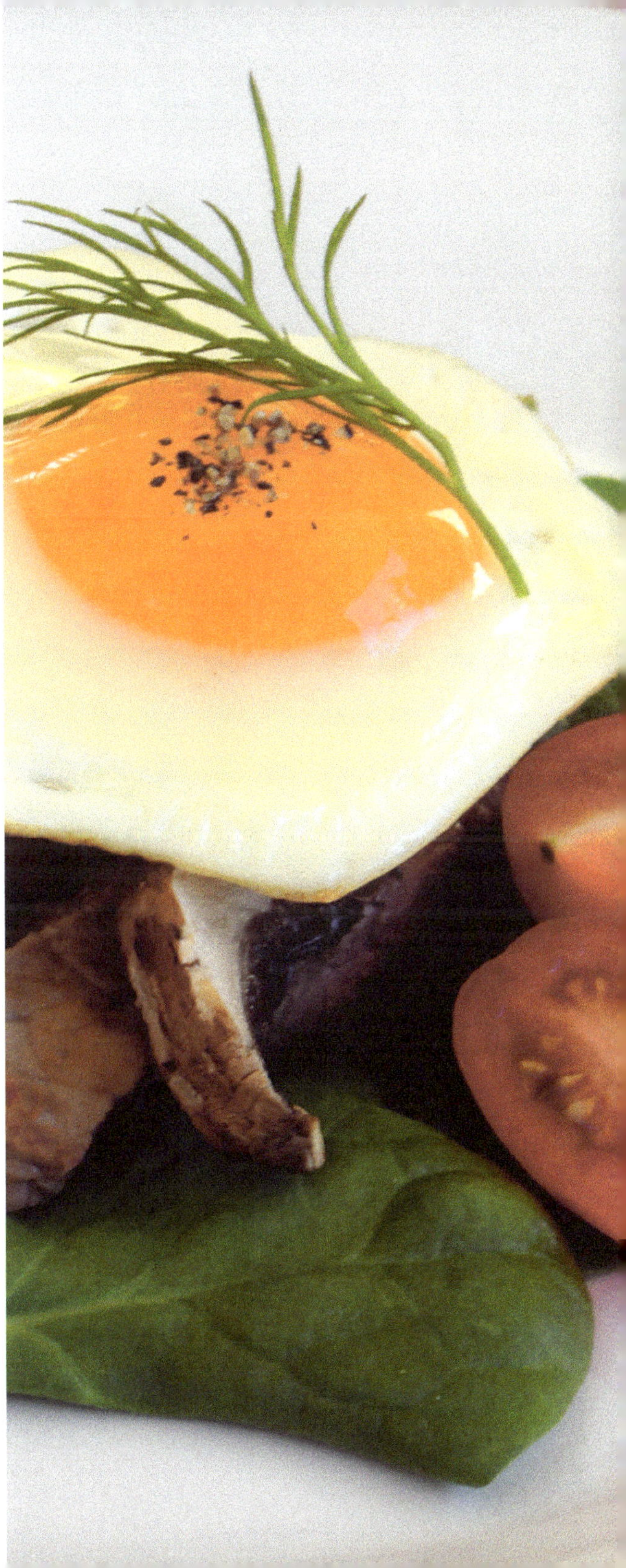

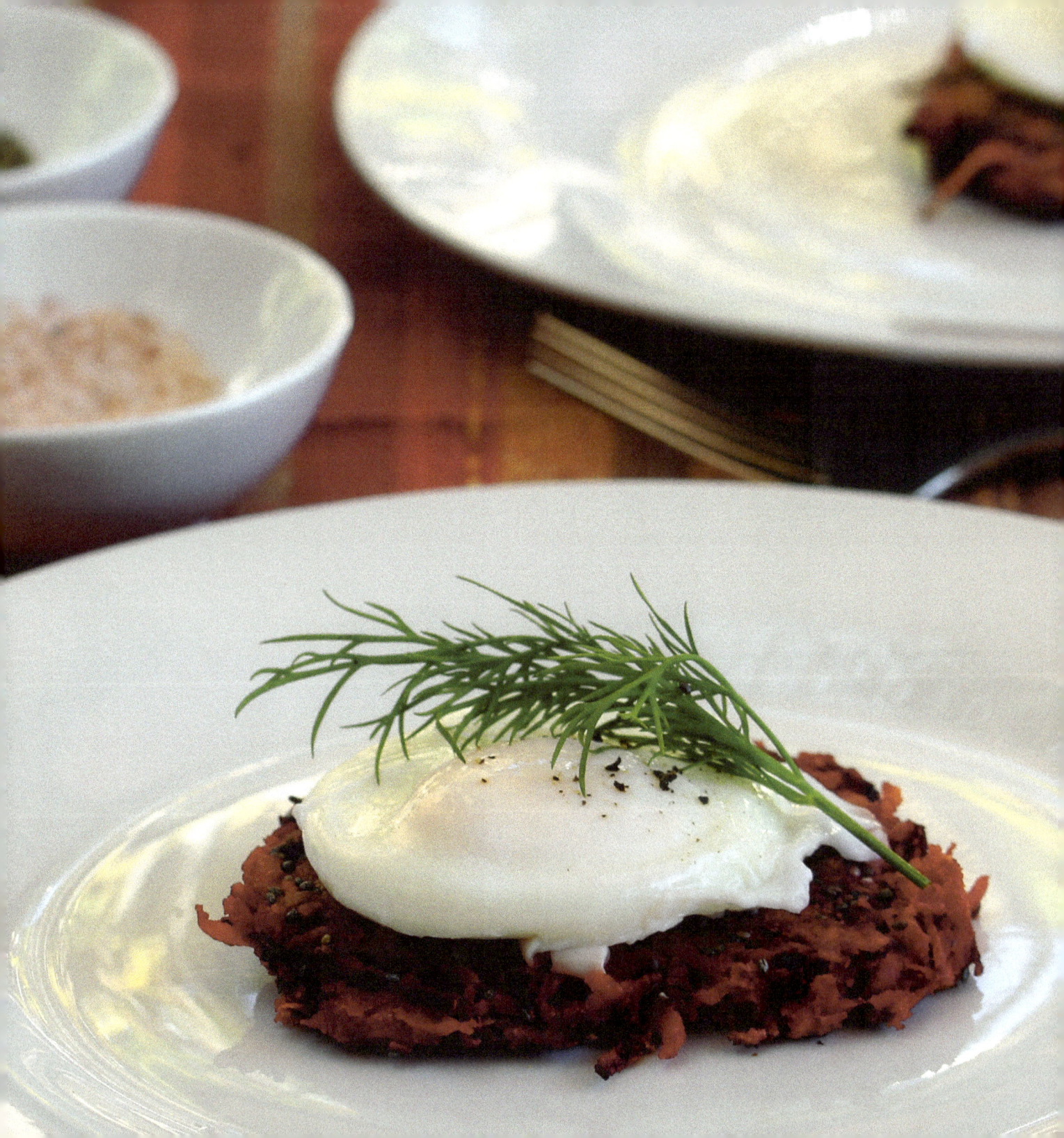

Poached eggs on sweet potato hash brown

Ingredients: 2 serves

3 eggs (1 for hash brown + 2 to poach)
1 cup of grated sweet potato
½ cup of grated Beetroot
¼ cup of coconut flour
½ diced onion (optional)
2 tablespoons of chia seeds
Pink mineral salt and cracked pepper to taste

Method:

Grate sweet potato and beetroot into a glass bowl. Add one egg, coconut flour, onion, chia seeds, pepper and salt and mix well. Heat a pan on low heat add 1 teaspoon of coconut oil and place a spoonful of mixture rolled into a ball into the pan and flatten into hash brown shape. Repeat with rest of the mixture. Cook on both sides for several minutes. While the hash browns are cooking poach the 2 remaining eggs.

Place another pan or pot on heat with 5cm-2inches of hot water and bring to simmer, and then add the two eggs cook for several minutes until egg white is solid. (Optional- a little apple cider vinegar can be added to poached egg water)

To plate up - place hash brown onto plate add poached egg on top garnish with a little fresh dill and cracked pepper. Fresh tomato can also be added as side serve.

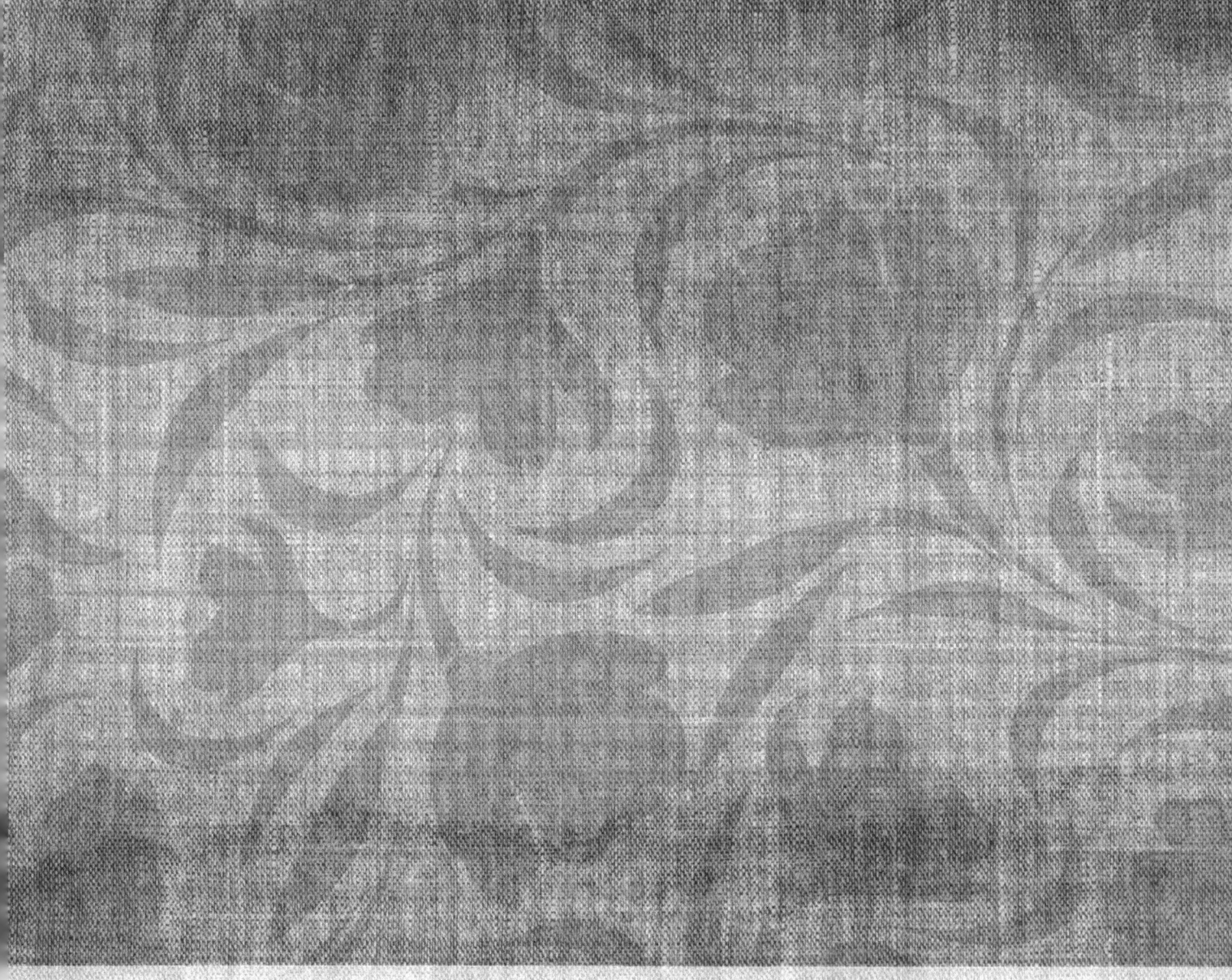

Nutritional yeast
Nutritional yeast is rich essential vitamins and minerals. It's one of the best non-animal sources of folic acid and vitamin B-12. The yellow colour of the flakes is a result of their large amount of vitamin B – ½ tablespoon fulfils your entire daily vitamin B needs. In addition to B-12, nutritional yeast is high in 15 different minerals and is a complete protein containing 18 amino acids. It is also naturally low in fat and sodium and is free of sugar, dairy, and gluten. Since it is plant derived and dried (out), it's free of the harmful candida that can wreak havoc on your digestive system.

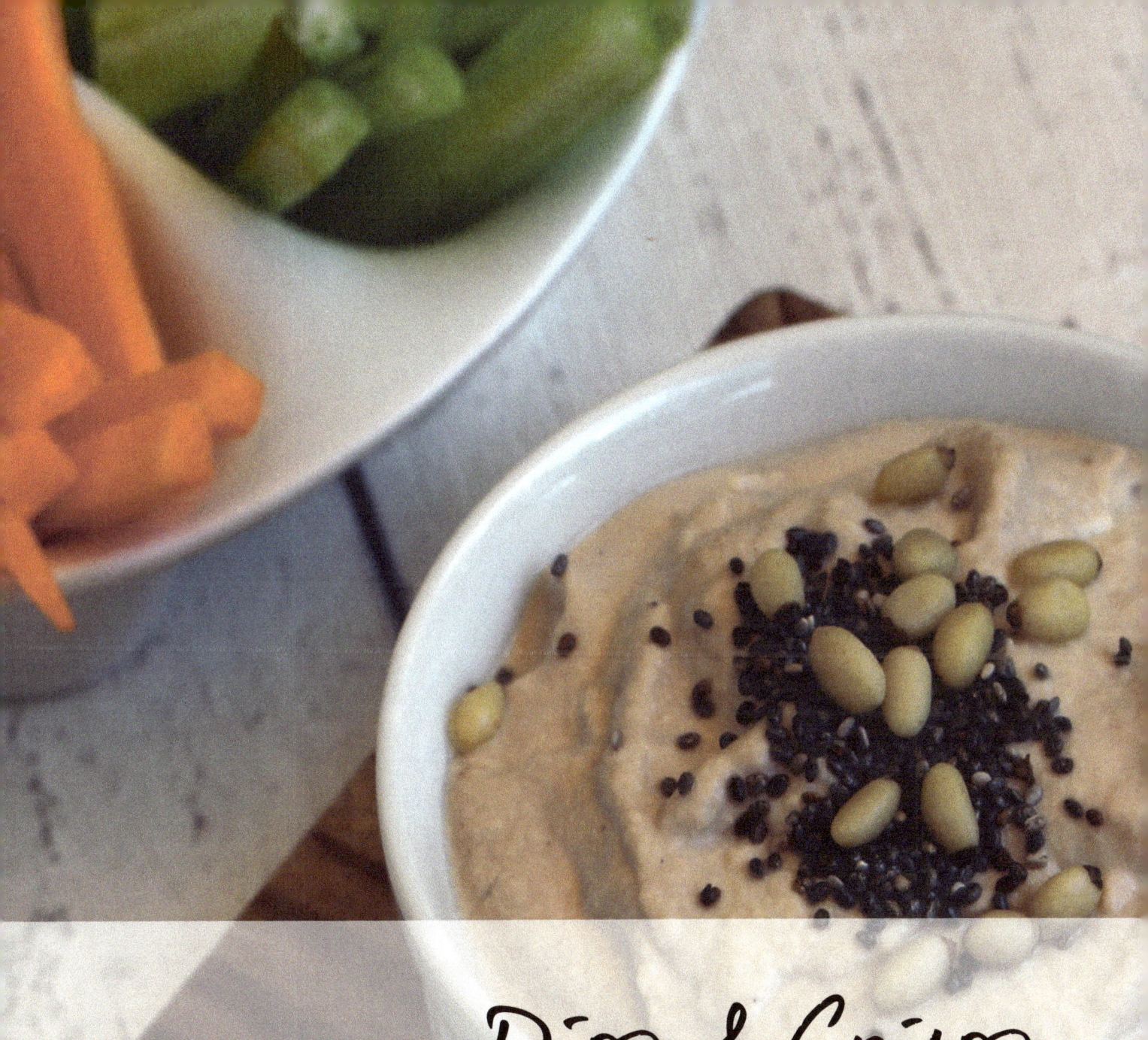

Dips & Crisps

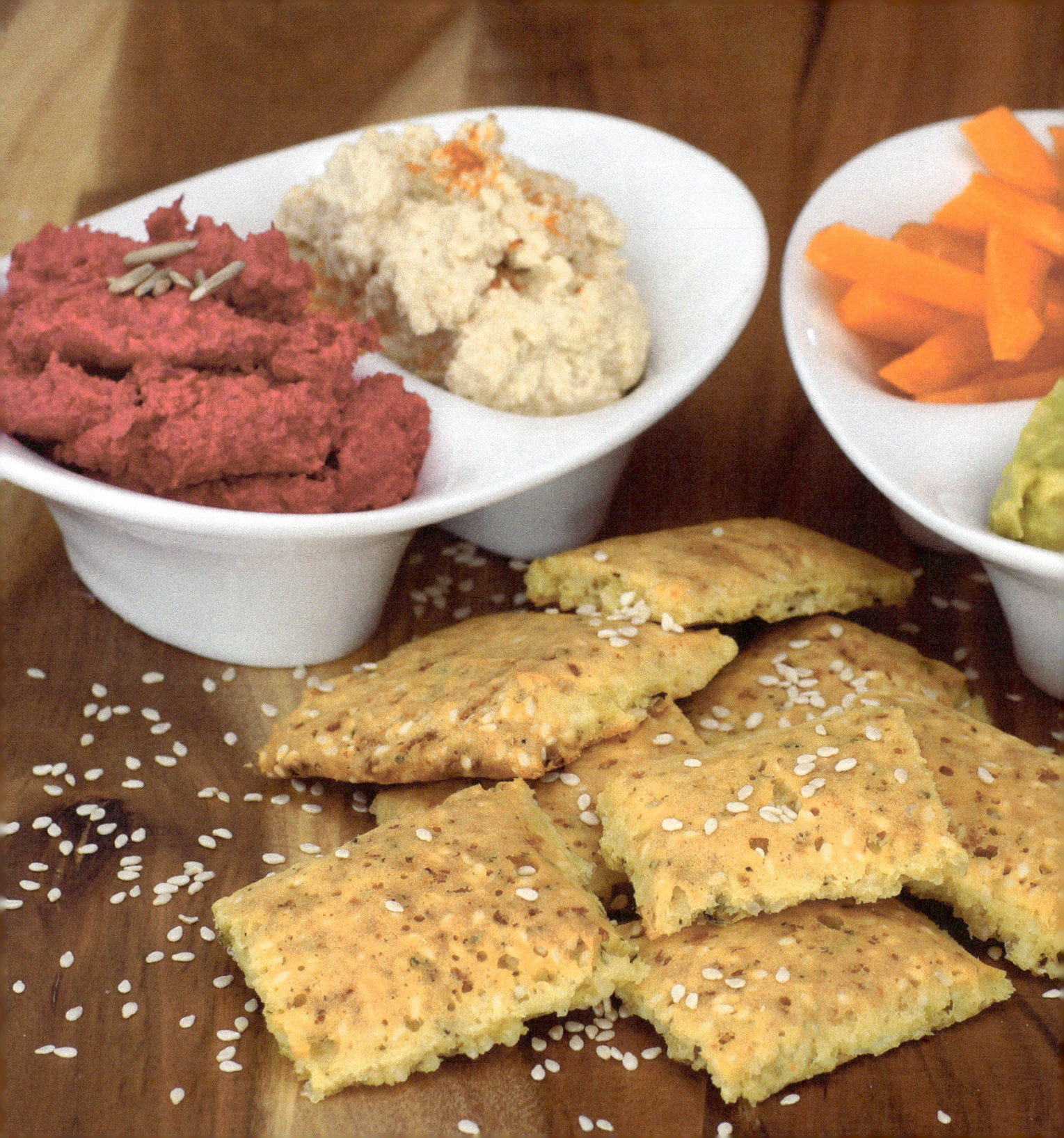

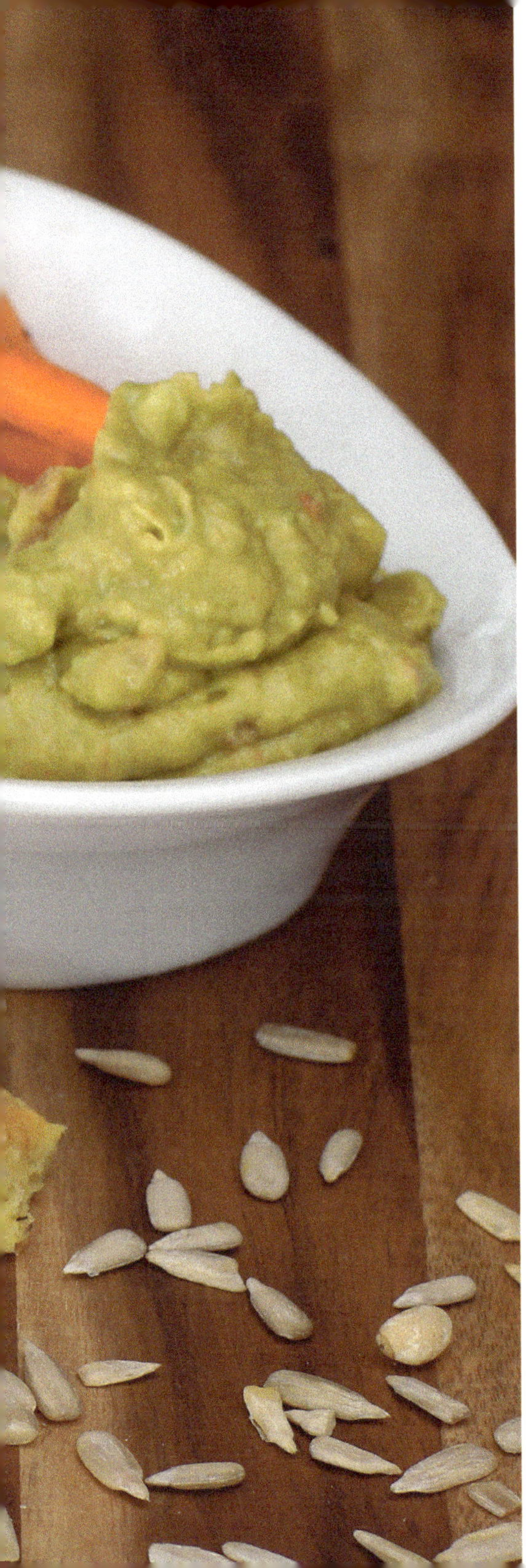

Spicy avocado

Ingredients:
2 soft avocados
1 ripe tomato
I small chopped red onion
2 teaspoons of extra virgin olive oil
Sprinkle of chilli to taste
Juice of one lemon
Season with Pinch of pink mineral salt & pepper to taste

Method:
Place all ingredients into blender and blend until smooth.
Taste and add more chilli as required. Garnish with chopped mix nuts (optional)

Beetroot dip

Ingredients:
2 medium or one large beetroot diced
Juice of one lemon
½ cup of cashews (activated optional)*
1 clove garlic
1/2 red onion diced
Pinch of pink mineral salt and pepper to taste
2 teaspoon of extra virgin olive oil
½ -1 cup of Coconut water as required to make a creamy texture

Method:
Place all ingredients into blender and blend until you have a soft thick texture, adding more coconut water as required.
Refrigerate in airtight container until ready to use.
*Activated cashews - soaked in salted water for a minimum 2-4 hours then drain.

Creamy tahini dip

Ingredients:
1 cup of sesame seeds
½ cup of cashew nuts (activated optional)*
1/4 of a cup extra virgin olive oil
2 cloves of minced garlic
½ cup of lemon juice
½-1 cup of filtered water (to achieve desired consistancy)
A sprinkle of paprika
½ teaspoon of nutritional yeast
Season with Pink mineral salt & cracked black pepper to taste

Method:
Place ingredients into a blender and blend until smooth, place in fridge in airtight container until ready to serve. Garnish with a dash of olive oil and a sprinkle of paprika.
*Activated cashews - soaked in salted water for a minimum 2-4 hours then drain.

Tangy Tomato salsa

Ingredients:

2 cups of diced tomatoes (4-6 tomatoes)
½ cup of diced cucumber
2 radishes diced finely
6 mustard seeds
½ teaspoon oregano
½ teaspoon basil
1 clove of garlic minced
½ juice of a lemon
½ juice of a lime
2 teaspoons of diced onion
½ a red chilli (you can add extra chilli for hot salsa)
½ teaspoon of turmeric powder (optional)
2 teaspoons of extra virgin olive oil
2 teaspoons of apple cider vinegar
Cracked black pepper & pinch of pink mineral salt to taste

Method:

Dice 4 tomatoes, cucumber, and radish and place in a bowl and set aside. Then add remainder 2 diced tomatoes, onion and all other ingredients into a blender and blend until creamy paste. Add this mixture to diced tomatoes, cucumber and radish and mix well. Store mixture in an airtight container in the fridge for 2 hours before serving. Serve with fresh vegetable sticks or nut crisps.

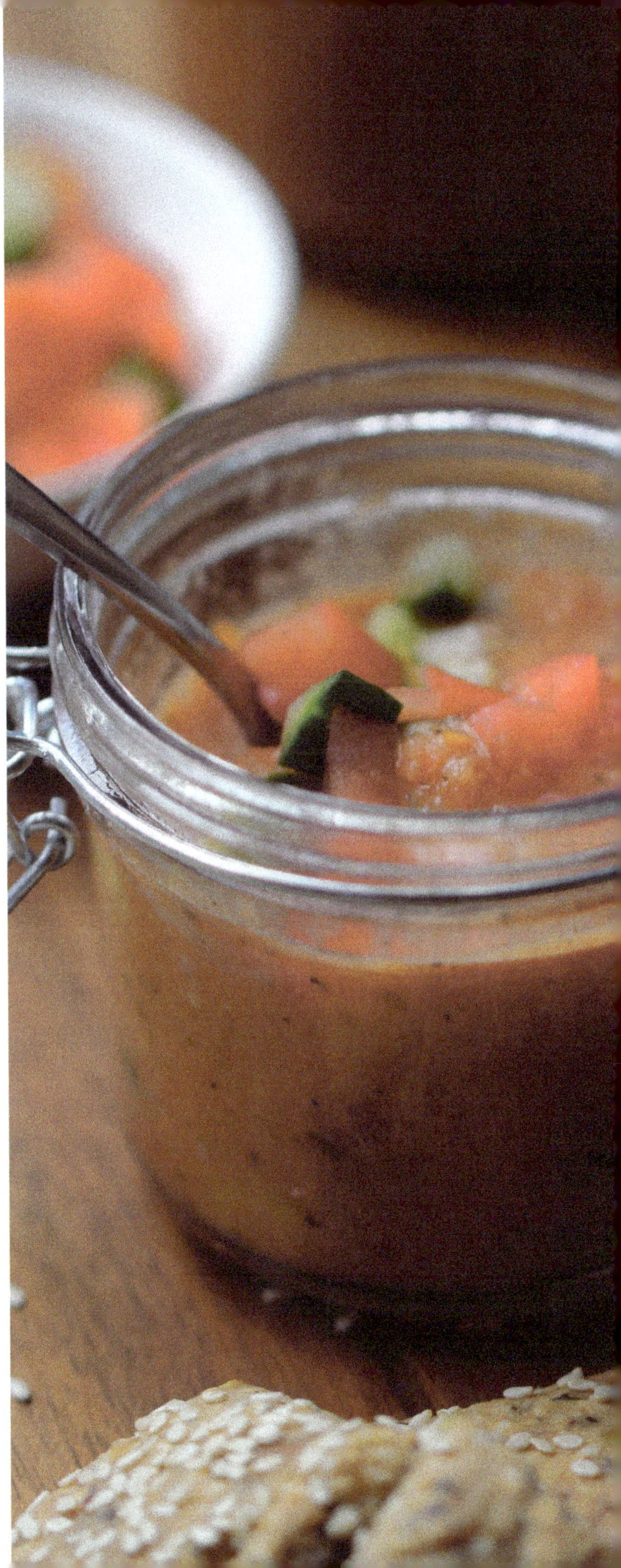

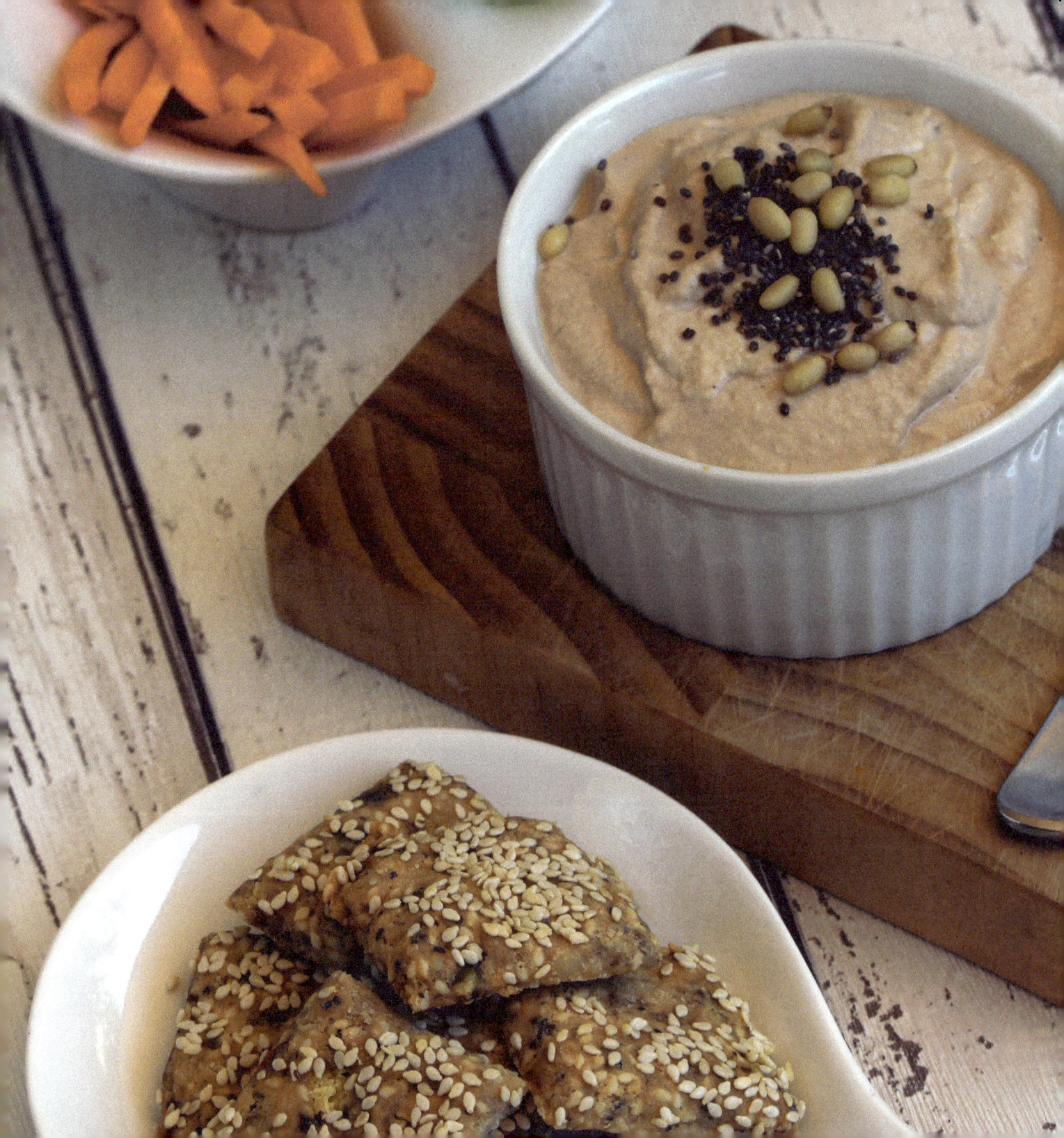

Salmon dip

Ingredients:
200 g of fresh cooked Atlantic salmon
(optional 210gm can drained pink salmon)
Juice of 2 lemons
½ cup of activated cashew nuts
Cracked black pepper to taste
½ teaspoon of nutritional yeast
(optional extra taste)
Pines nuts to garnish

Method:
Place activated nuts into the blender with juice of one lemon and blend until smooth adding extra lemon juice to taste. Then add salmon, onion and juice of second lemon and blend for another 10 -15 seconds until a smooth paste. Place in fridge to chill. Serve Topped with diced spring onions or pine nuts and chia seeds. Eat the same day.
*Activated cashews - soaked in salted water for a minimum 2-4 hours then drain.

Sesame seed chia crisps

Ingredients:
½ cup of sesame seeds (or flax seeds)
1½ cups of hazelnut meal or Almond meal
¼ cup pepitas (pumpkin seeds)
2 tablespoons of chia seeds
½ cup of chopped mix nuts*
2 eggs
Sprinkle of oregano and basil
1 teaspoon of nutritional yeast
Pinch of pink mineral salt (optional)
Cracked black pepper to taste
¼ cup of Coconut oil

Method:
Place all dry ingredients into a glass bowl mix in eggs and then coconut oil. Place mixture on to a flat baking tray lined with baking paper. Place another sheet of baking paper over the top of the mixture and roll mixture out thinly, remove top layer of paper and sprinkle extra sesame seeds on top. Score lines horizontal and vertical through the mixture with knife. Bake in oven heated to 165 degrees for 15-20 minutes or until golden brown. Remove and cool on cooling rack. Break into small squares, store in an airtight container in the fridge.
*cashews, walnuts, almonds, hazelnuts, pistachios, and macadamias

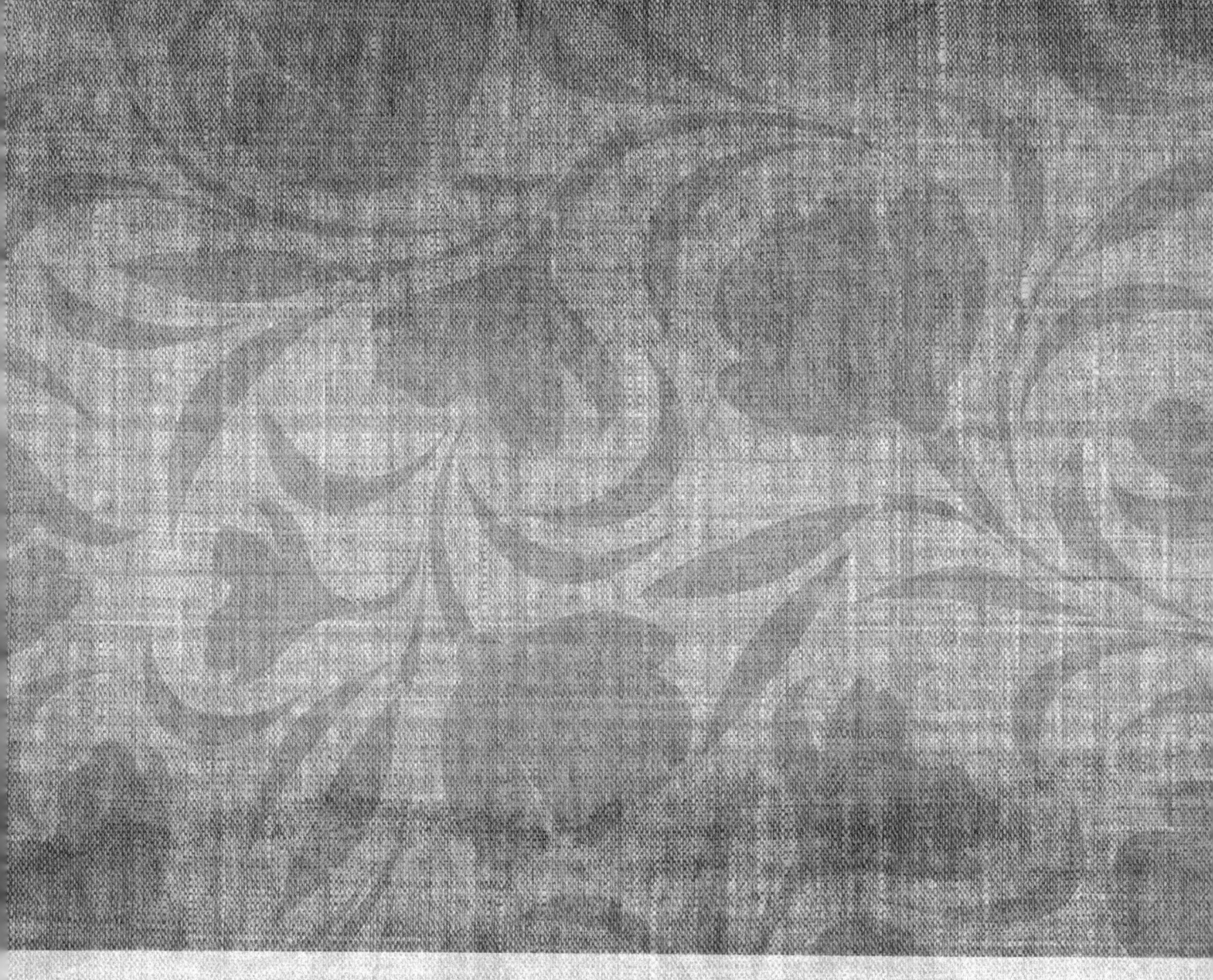

The benefits of turmeric

Turmeric contains carbohydrates, fibre, and is a complete protein, providing all nine essential amino acids. It is also a source of selenium and potassium. Turmeric contains curcumin which has powerful anti-inflammatory effects, antitumor, antibacterial, and antiviral activities and is a very strong antioxidant.

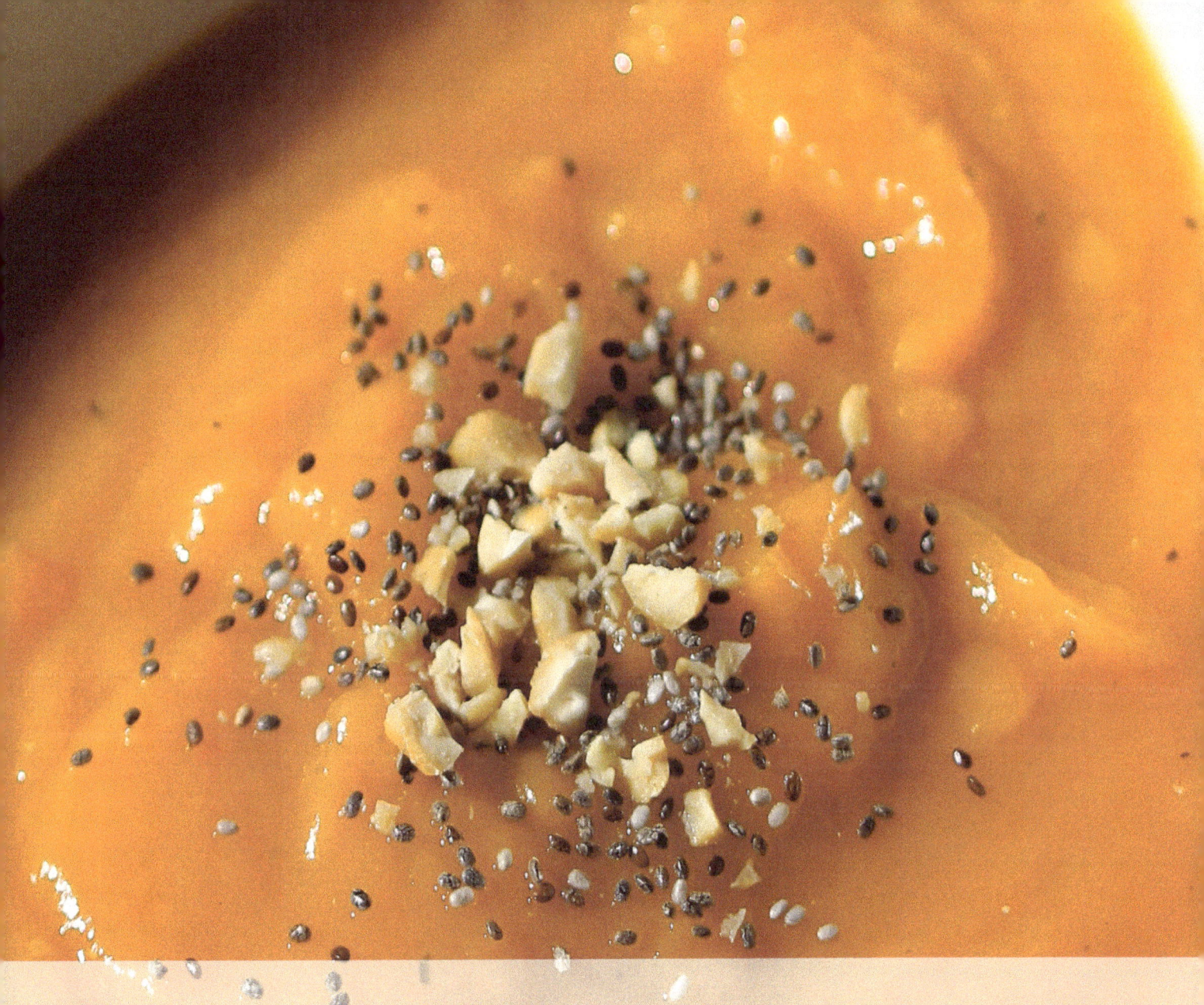

Soups

Pumpkin soup

Ingredients: 2-4 Serves

¼ of a jap pumpkin or ½ a butternut pumpkin
½ red onion diced
1-2 cloves of garlic (finely sliced)
1 teaspoon of fresh ginger (finely sliced)
1 dessertspoon of coconut oil
1 teaspoon of cinnamon
½ a diced chilli or sprinkle of chilli powder (adjust to your taste)
Filtered water
A pinch of pink mineral salt and cracked pepper to taste.
Garnish each bowl with 1 teaspoon of chia seeds, slivered almonds, or cashew nuts.

Method:

Place coconut oil into pot on low to medium heat, then add ginger, onion and garlic and stir occasionally for several minutes. Then take off the heat and add pumpkin and filtered water (to just cover the pumpkin), salt and pepper and place back on the heat, cover with lid and slowly bring just to a simmer for 5 minutes. Then turn off and let stand for 15 minutes. Place all contents of you pot into a blender and blend until a smooth consistency, serve and garnish with almond slithers, chia seeds or finely chopped cashew nuts.

A quick and easy soup. You can also add carrot or broccoli for a change.

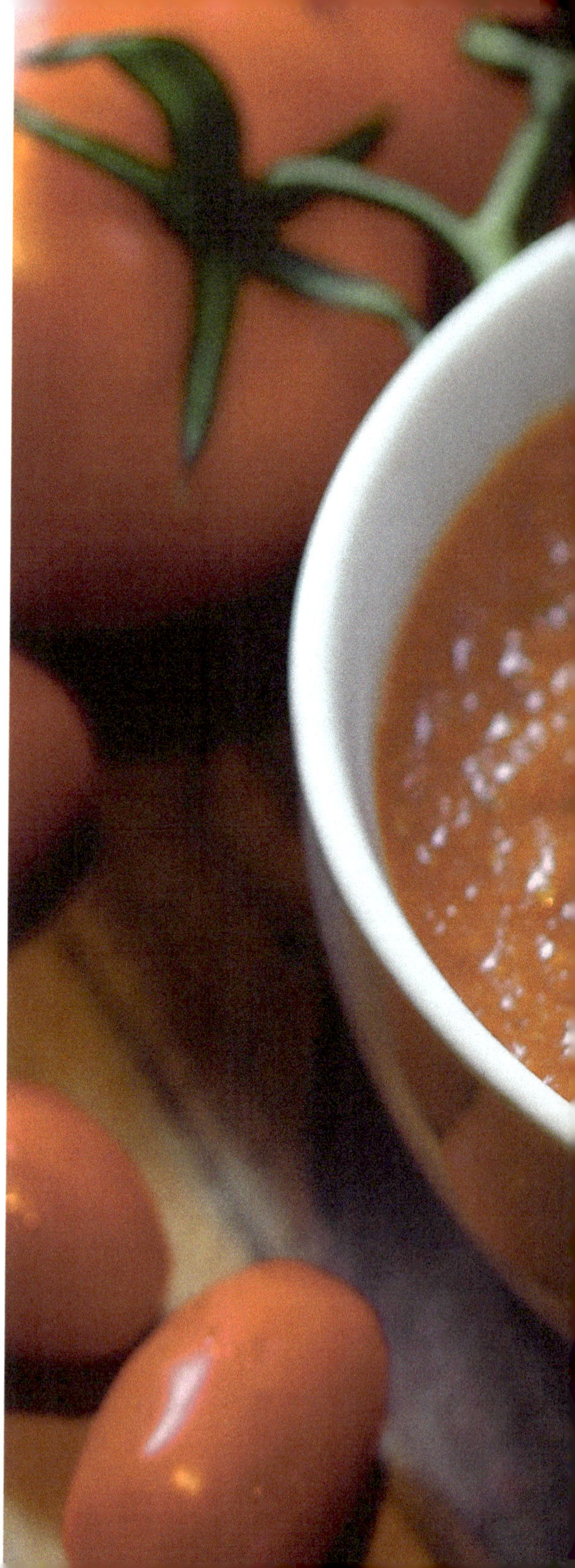

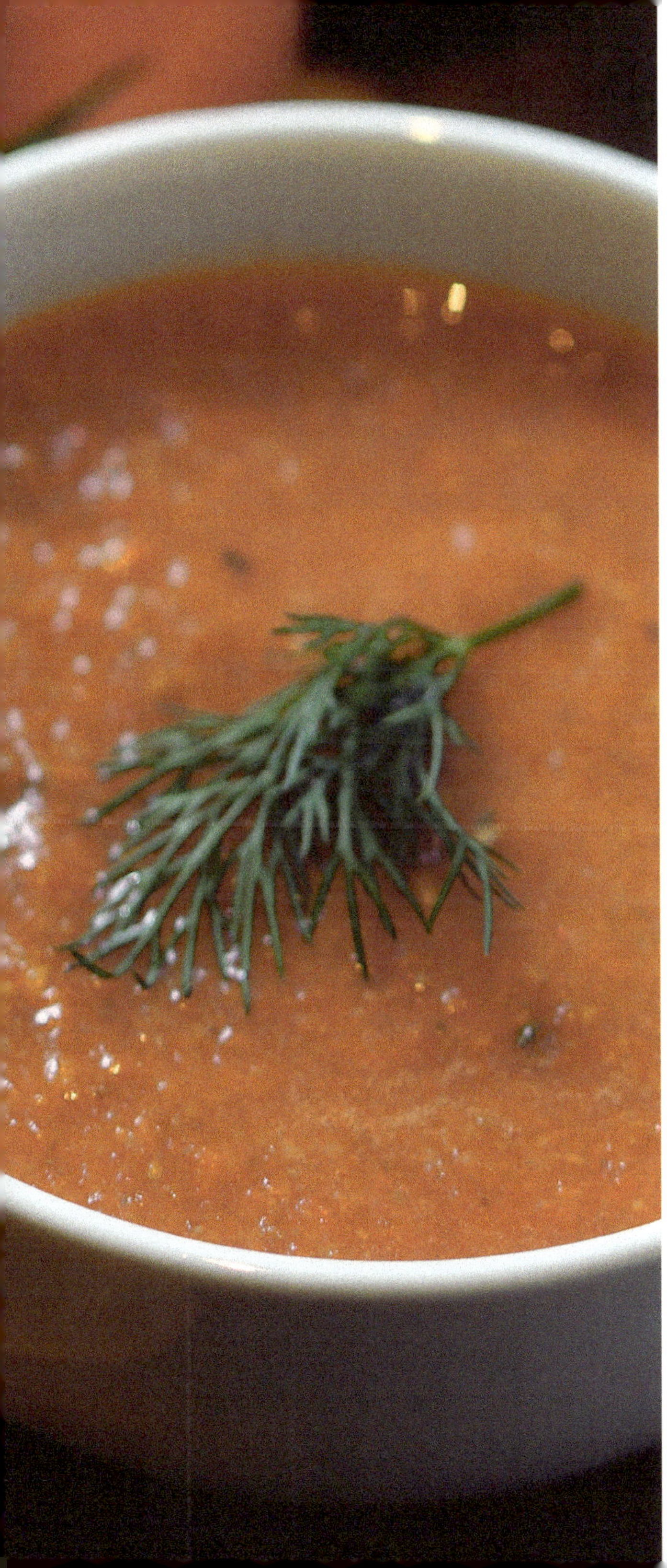

Tomato soup

Ingredients: 4 serves

1kg ripe tomatoes diced
4 sliced mushrooms
2 teaspoons of coconut oil
2 cloves of garlic diced
½ fresh chilli or chilli powder (optional)
1 teaspoon of turmeric powder
1 teaspoon of cumin
½ red onion
1 cup of coconut water (filtered water can be used as alternative)
1 cup coconut milk
Pink mineral salt and pepper to taste
Fresh basil garnish (optional)

Method:

Place coconut oil into a pot on a medium heat, add onion, garlic, turmeric, chilli and cumin and stir for a few minutes to release aromas and onion is clear. Then add pureed tomatoes, diced mushrooms, salt and pepper and 1 cup of coconut water. Simmer for 20 minutes until soup thickens adding more water if needed. Serve garnished with a sprinkle of fresh basil optional. For finer texture blend soup in blender for 15 seconds and serve.

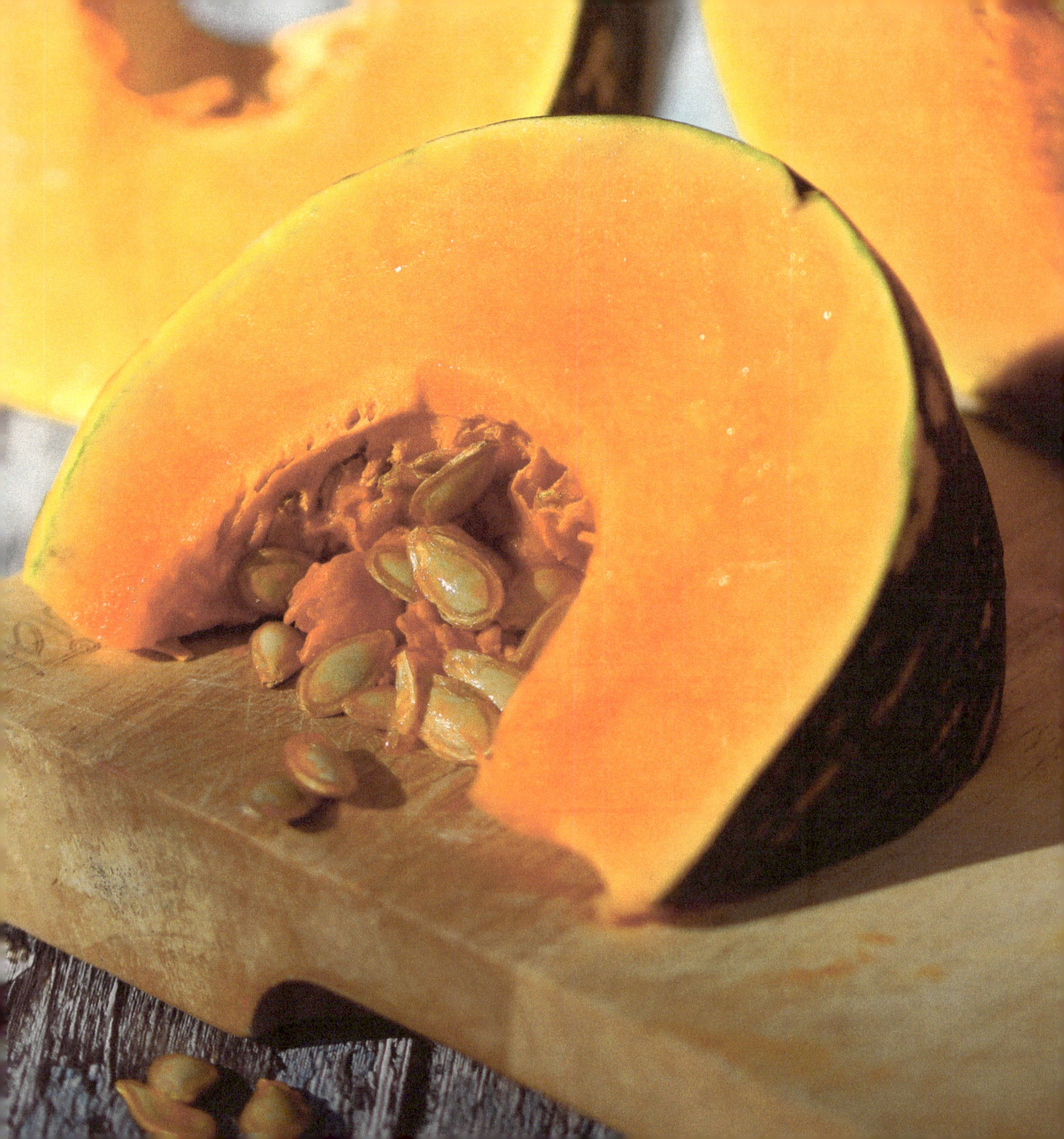

Vegetable soup

Ingredients: 2-4 sevres

4 cups of cubed pumpkin

1 red onion diced

2 cloves garlic

2 cups broccoli chopped

1 cup of sweet potato cubed

2 cups spinach

½ egg plant cubed

5 tomatoes

3 zucchinis cubed

1 teaspoon ginger

1 teaspoon turmeric ground

1 teaspoon cumin ground

1 teaspoon cinnamon ground

½ teaspoon chilli powder (optional)

1 teaspoon of dried oregano

1 teaspoon of dried basil

Fresh basil to garnish

Method:

Wash all vegetables in filtered water dice into cubes. Place a large soup pot on a medium heat add coconut oil, diced onion, garlic and cook until onion is clear, then add all herbs and spices for a minute or two to release the flavours.

Finally add vegetables (except spinach) and add water just almost cover vegetables, then add tomatoes and place a lid on the pot and cook on low heat (just simmer) for 10 minutes then add spinach and turn the heat off and leave to stand with the lid on for another 15 minutes. Serve and garnish with fresh basil or alternatively place in the blender and puree' for 20 seconds and serve. Garnish with fresh basil and a sprinkle of nutritional yeast.

Lamb & pumpkin soup

Ingredients: 2-4 serves

200 grams cubed lamb* (14.11 ounces)
4 cups cubed pumpkin
1 red onion diced
1 clove of garlic crushed
1 teaspoon of ginger grated
1 teaspoon of turmeric powder
1 pinch of pink mineral salt and pepper to taste
2 dessertspoons coconut oil
2 cups of coconut milk
Filtered water as required
Coriander and pine nuts to garnish

Method:

Place coconut oil into a pan and cook lamb in batches (6 pieces at a time) for several minutes until brown and place aside. Place a large soup pot on medium heat and add 1 dessertspoon of coconut oil, onion, garlic ginger and turmeric powder and cook for a few minutes until onion is clear. Then add tomatoes browned lamb and coconut milk, pepper and salt and cover. Simmer on low heat for 40 minutes. Add pumpkin and filtered water as required if too thick. Simmer for another 20 minutes until pumpkin and lamb are cooked.
Garnish with fresh coriander and pine nuts.
*Chicken can be used instead of Lamb

Spicy thai soup

Ingredients: 2-4 serves

1 large celery stick
1 medium carrot
2 cups of coconut water
2 cups water
1/4 cup of cashews
1 clove of garlic
1 spring onion
½ a capsicum
½ a lime
1 teaspoon ginger
½ a chilli
½ cup fresh coriander
Pinch of pink mineral salt
Cracked pepper to taste
Chicken shredded (high protein option)

Method:

Place all ingredients into blender and blend for 3-5 minutes for instant soup. Garnish with fresh coriander and add shredded chicken meat for a high protein optional extra. If your blender does not heat the soup place in a pot on low heat until warmed through.

Broccoli spinach soup

Ingredients: 2-4 serves

3 cups fresh broccoli
3 cups of fresh spinach leaves
2 zucchini diced
½ cup of fresh parsley, roughly chopped
2 tablespoons of sauerkraut
1 dessertspoon of coconut oil
2 cloves of garlic, chopped
1 diced red onion
2 teaspoons of fresh ginger, chopped finely
½ a small chilli diced (optional)
½ teaspoon of turmeric (optional)
Sprinkle of dried basil
Pinch of pink mineral salt and ground pepper
squeeze of fresh lemon juice
Fresh filtered water, as needed

Method:

Using a large soup pot, heat the coconut oil over medium heat and stir in the garlic, onion, and ginger to season the oil. Add the broccoli, zucchini, and parsley, and then add just enough water to almost cover the vegetables. You can always add more water later to thin the soup if needed. Bring to a low simmer, cover the pot, and simmer low for 5 minutes and turn heat off and add spinach and sauerkraut let stand for 10 minutes. Place mixture into a blender and puree the soup. Adding a little more lemon juice if required. Garnish with chopped cashew nuts or fresh basil.

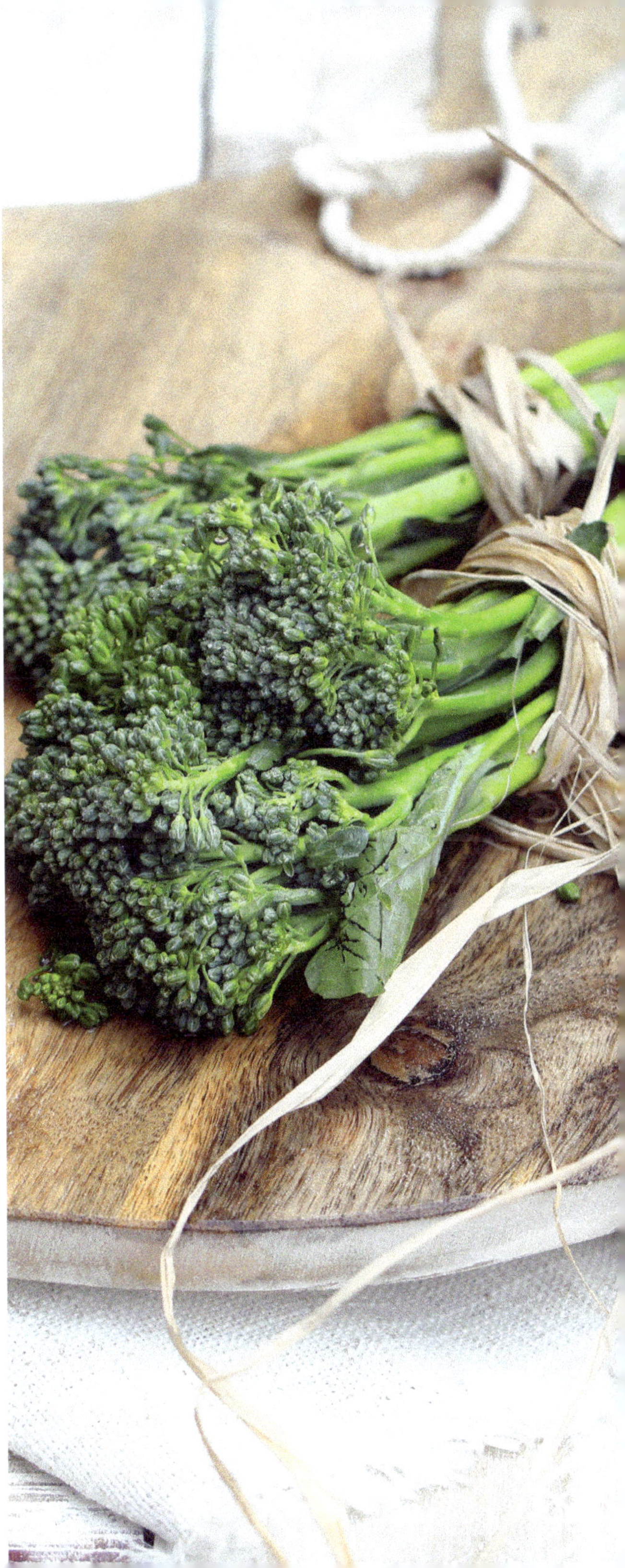

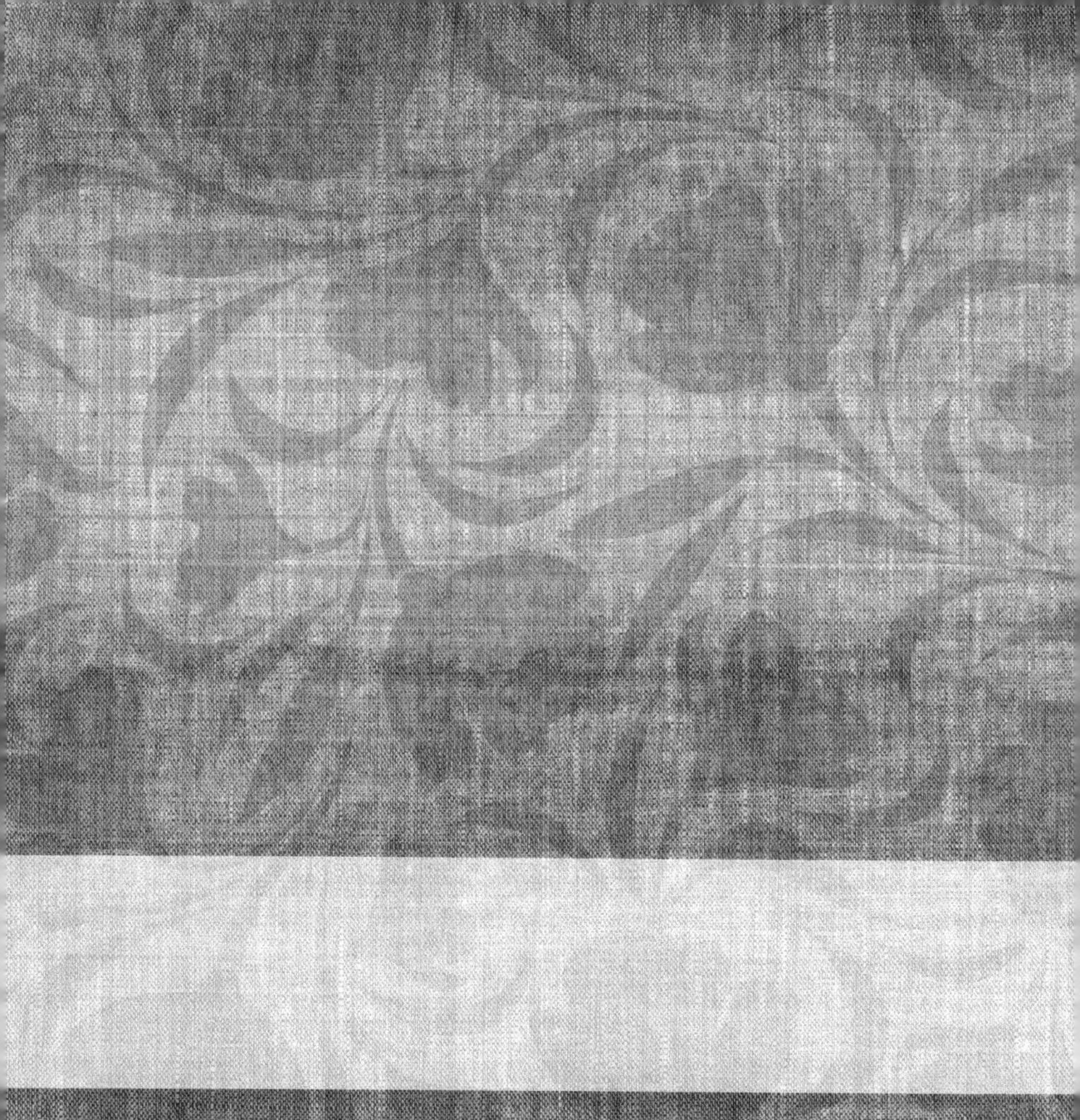

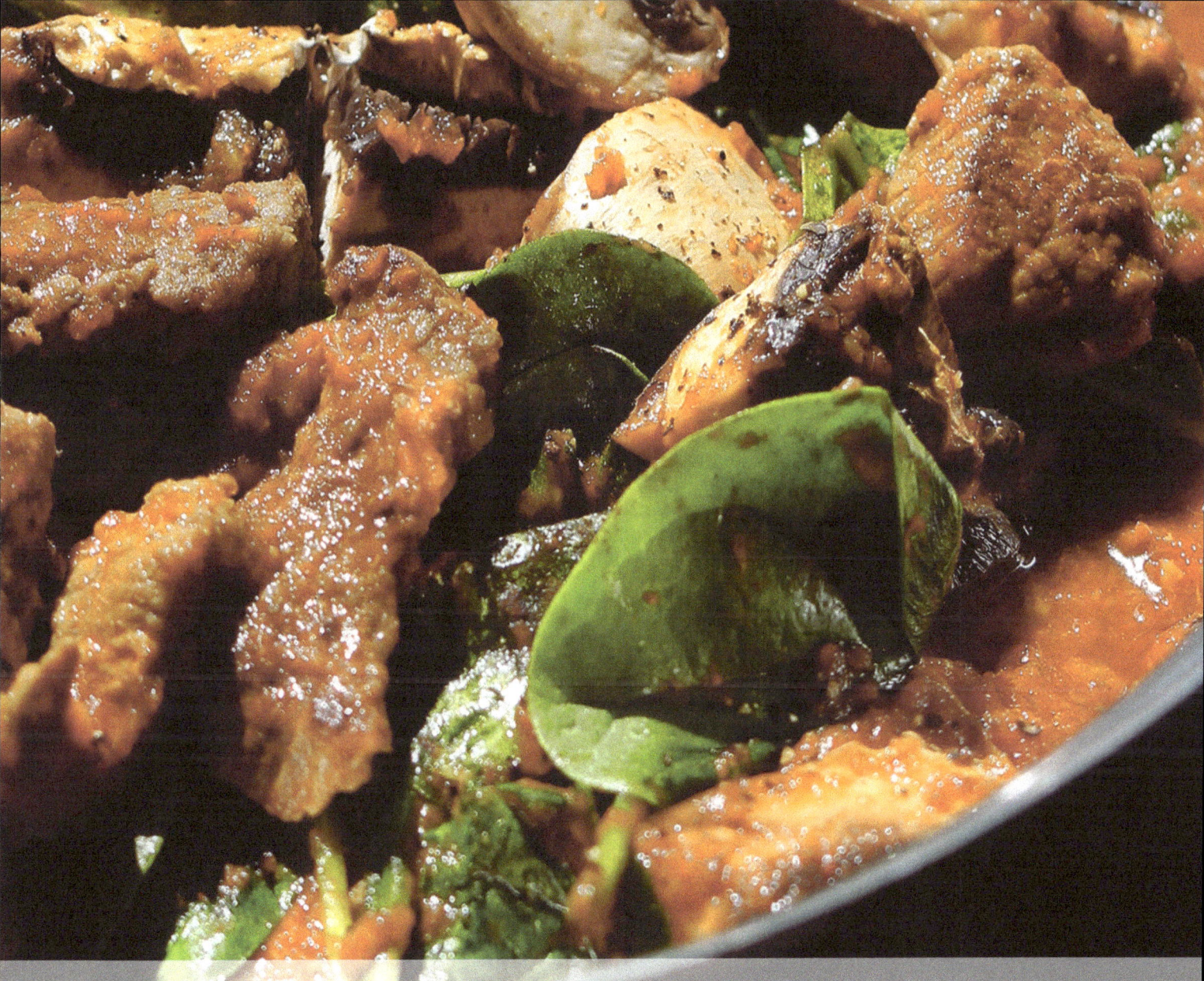

Dinner

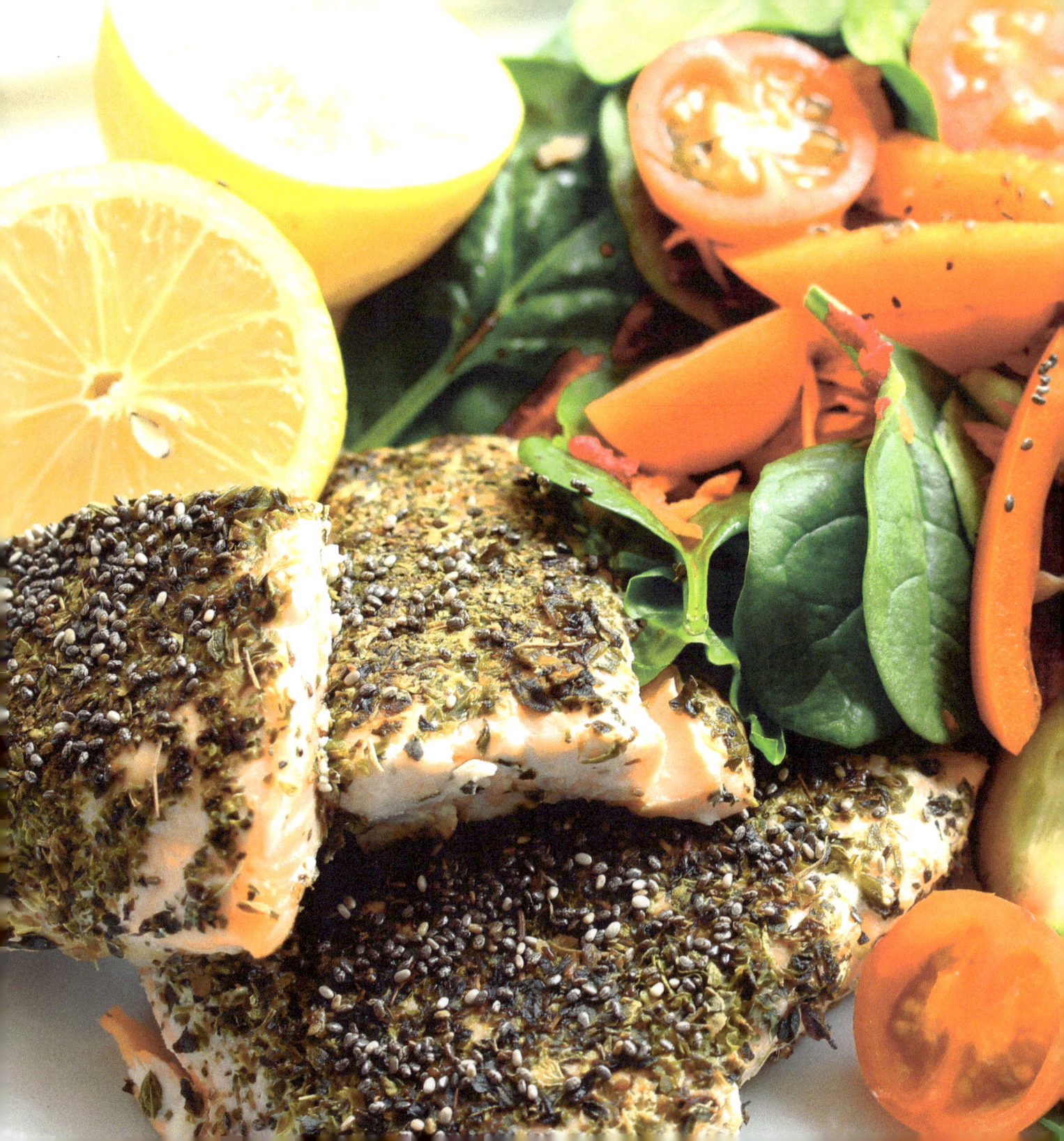

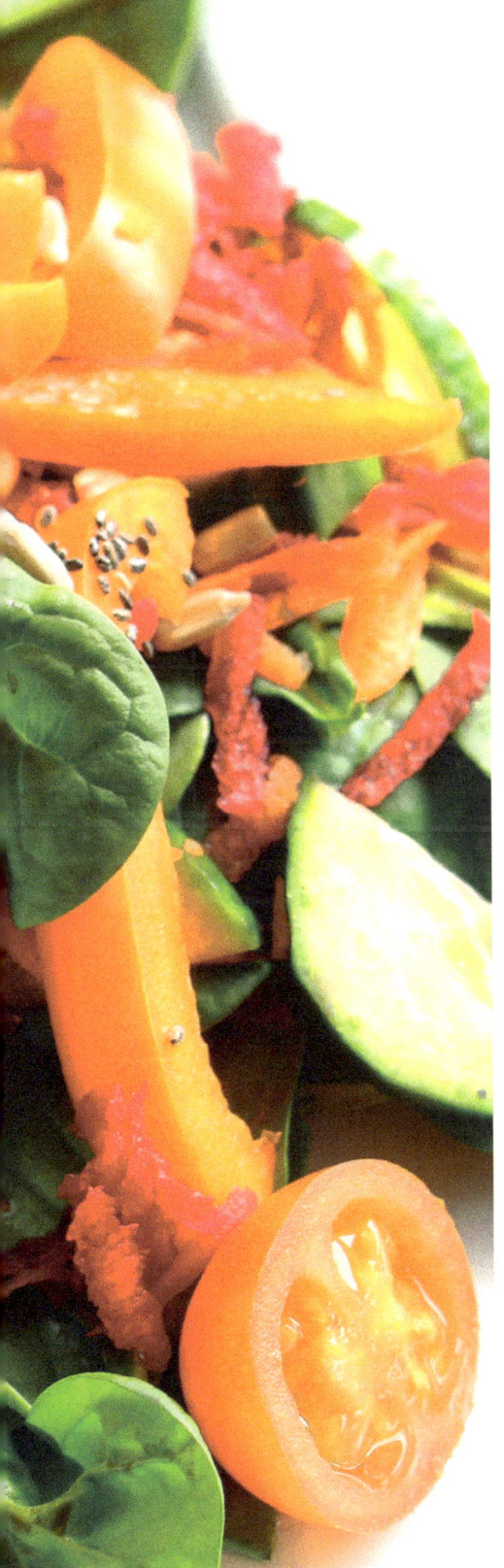

Atlantic salmon and salad

Ingredients: 2 serves

Two serves of Atlantic salmon (2 x 100 gams)
1 teaspoon of coconut oil
Coriander ground
Chia seeds
Basil ground
Baby spinach leaves
Cherry tomatoes
Cucumber sliced
Grated or spiraled carrot
Grated or spiraled Beetroot
Thinly sliced radish
Juice of one lemon
Sprinkle of chia seeds to garnish salad optional

Method:

Place pan on low to medium heat with a little coconut oil then add the Atlantic salmon coated with coriander, chia seeds and basil and add to the pan. Cook on low medium heat. While salmon is cooking prepare the salad. Wash the baby spinach leaves and drain well, add cherry tomatoes, cucumber, radish, carrot and beetroot. Then plate up the salmon and dress salad with lemon juice or one of my salad dressing recipes:
 Mustard-orange garlic salad dressing, or lemon-herb dressing, or apple cider vinegar-mustard vinaigrette.

Prawns on zucchini pasta

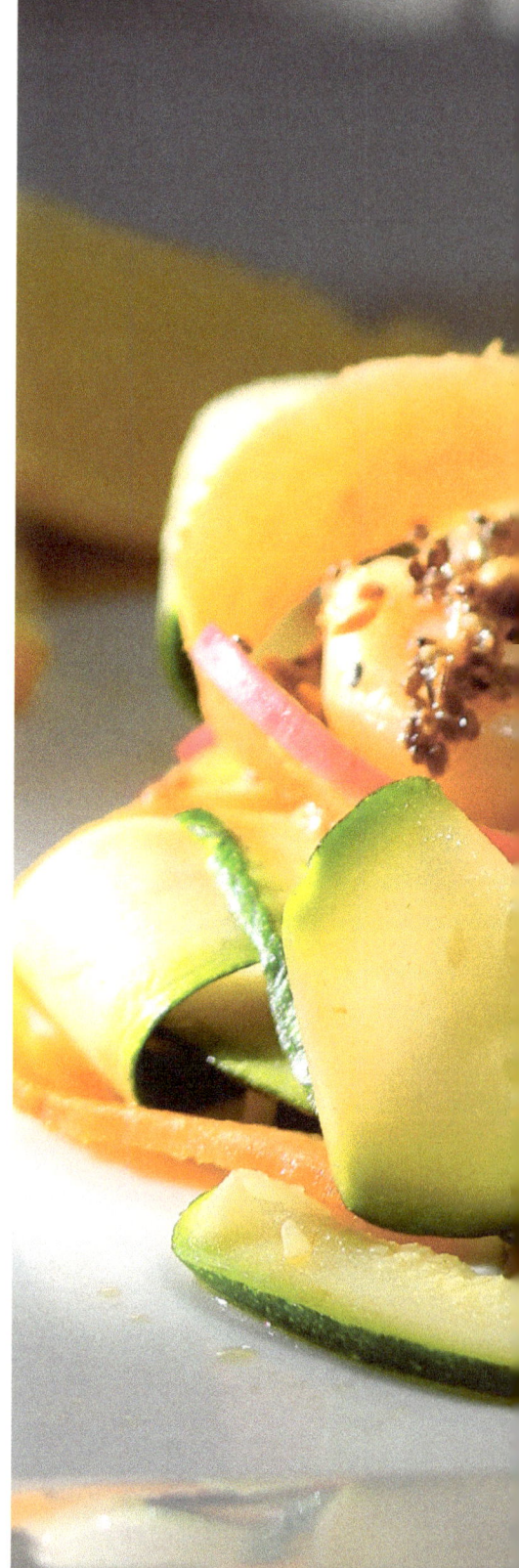

Ingredients: 2-4 serves

12 green Prawns
2 zucchinis
3 radishes
1 carrot
1 red capsicum
Juice of 2 lemons
1 clove garlic

1 teaspoon of cumin seeds
1 teaspoon of coriander seeds
1 teaspoon of fennel seed
1 teaspoon of mustard seeds
1 dessertspoon of chia seeds
2 dessertspoons Coconut oil
2 tablespoons of extra virgin olive oil
Black pepper and pink mineral salt to taste

Method:

Heat pan on medium heat and add cumin, fennel, and coriander, and mustard seeds and stirring constantly for a few minutes until you can smell the aroma of the spices. Then place them into a mortar or spice grinder and grind to fine powder. Then place powder into a glass bowl with crushed garlic, dessertspoon of coconut oil, chia seeds and juice of one lemon mix well. Coat the prawns well and place in the fridge for 15 minutes to marinate. Take the zucchinis and carrot, using a vegetable peeler cut into long thin ribbons. Slice the radishes and red capsicum very finely and add to a bowl with pepper, salt, juice of one lemon and olive oil, toss vegetables gently. Next heat pan on low to medium heat add 1 dessertspoon of coconut oil and cook prawns for a couple of minutes until they go pink. Then add to vegetable pasta and serve.

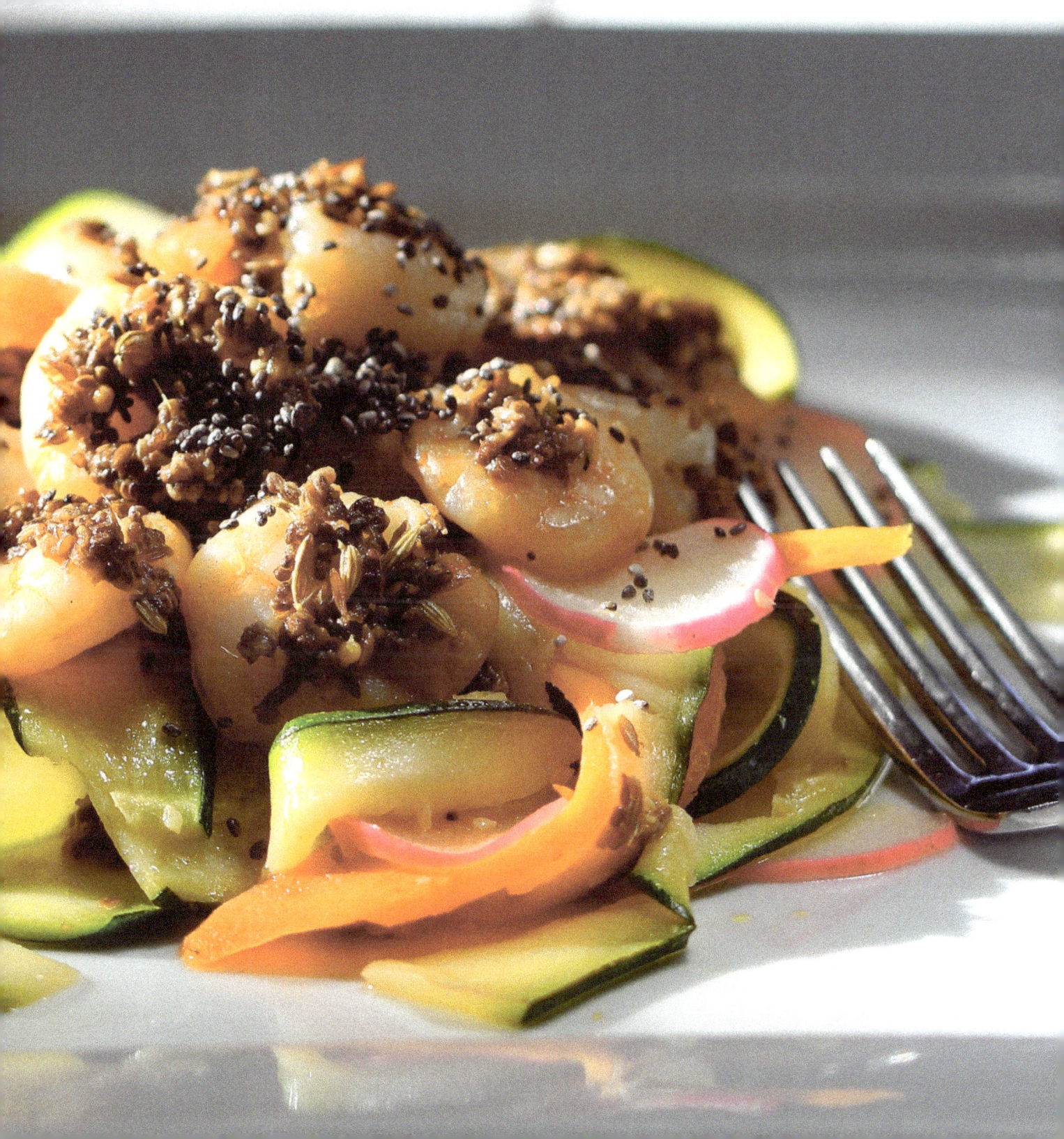

Roasted chicken breast on cauliflower purée

Ingredients: 2 serves

2 chicken breasts
1 cup of Almond meal (for coating chicken)
Coconut oil for basting
1 teaspoon of chilli flakes or paprika (mild flavour)
1 teaspoon of grounded cumin seeds
1 clove of garlic finely diced
1 teaspoon of grated ginger
Season with pink mineral salt and cracked pepper
1 teaspoon of nutritional yeast (optional extra flavour)
½ head of cauliflower grated
2 serves of broccoli
2 serves of pumpkin

Method:

Preheat your oven to 180 degrees Celsius /175 fan forced. Place almond meal in a deep glass bowl with chilli flakes, cumin powder; garlic diced, grated ginger, salt and pepper mix well. Then baste the chicken with a little coconut oil and roll into crumb mixture coating the chicken breasts well. Place chicken into glass oven proof dish and sprinkle lightly with nutritional yeast (optional). Bake in the oven for 20-25 minutes.

Cauliflower purée

Grate ½ a head of raw cauliflower into an oven proof glass bowl. Season with salt (pink) and fresh cracked pepper and a little nutritional yeast and mix well. Place the bowl covered with a lid over a pot of hot water and steam lightly for 4 minutes until mixture is hot then put mixture into a blender and blend until pureed. Adding a little filtered water if needed.

Broccoli and pumpkin

Chop broccoli and pumpkin into small pieces baste pumpkin with a little coconut oil, and bake in the oven for the same amount of time as the chicken, adding the broccoli for the last ten minutes.
Alternatively lightly steam pumpkin and broccoli four several minutes.

Plating up

Place the puree on the plate then place the chicken breast on top and serve pumpkin and broccoli on the side. Heated home make tomato sauce can be added on top for those who enjoy their sauces.

Beef/chicken strips with tomato and spinach

Ingredients: 2 serves

200-400grams of beef or chicken strips
1 cup baby spinach leaves
1-2 cups homemade tomato sauce*
3 mushrooms or capsicum diced
1 clove crushed garlic (optional)
1 teaspoon cumin ground powder
1 teaspoon of cinnamon powder
Fresh chilli or chilli ground powder
1 teaspoon of coconut oil

Method:

Place pan on low to medium heat with coconut oil, then add garlic, chilli and cook for one minute add meat, cumin, cinnamon and cook until brown, mixing spices with the meat. Once meat is browned, then add tomato sauce, mushrooms and simmer for a further 2 minutes finally add spinach leaves to mixture and serve.

*homemade tomato sauce under sauces section

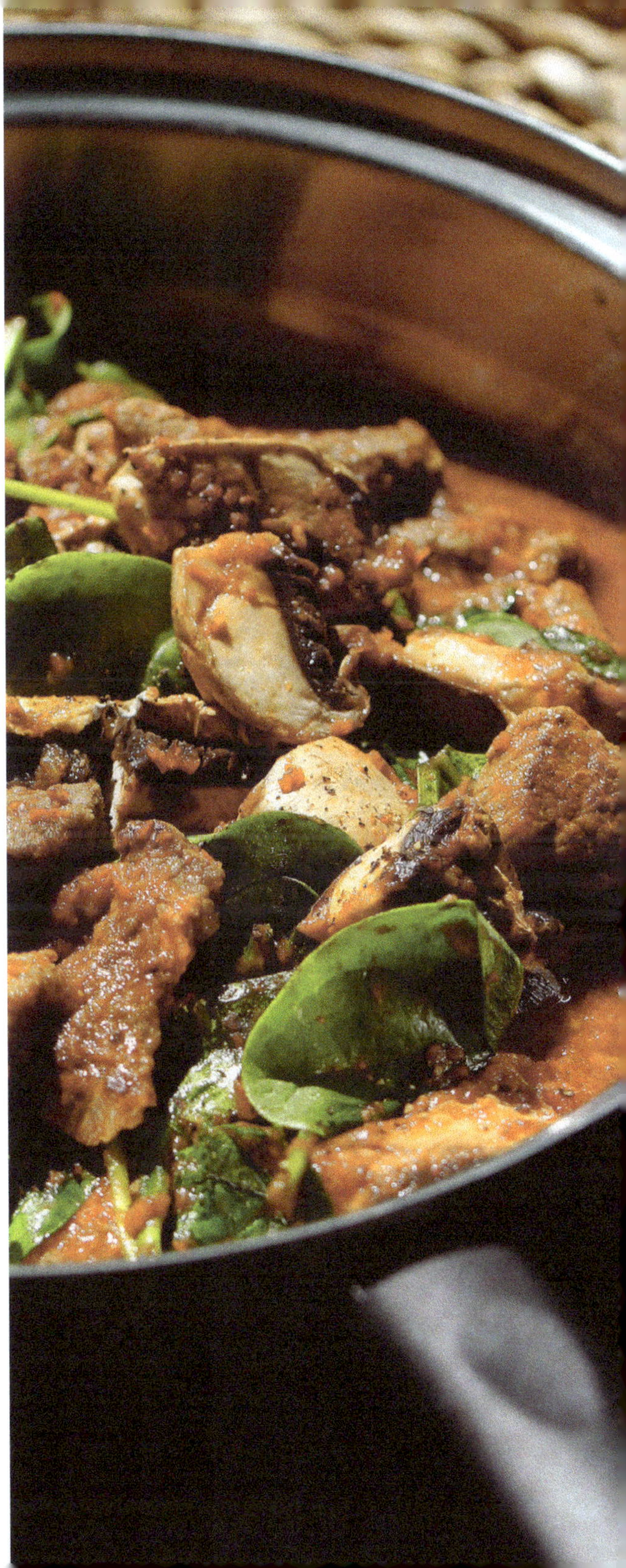

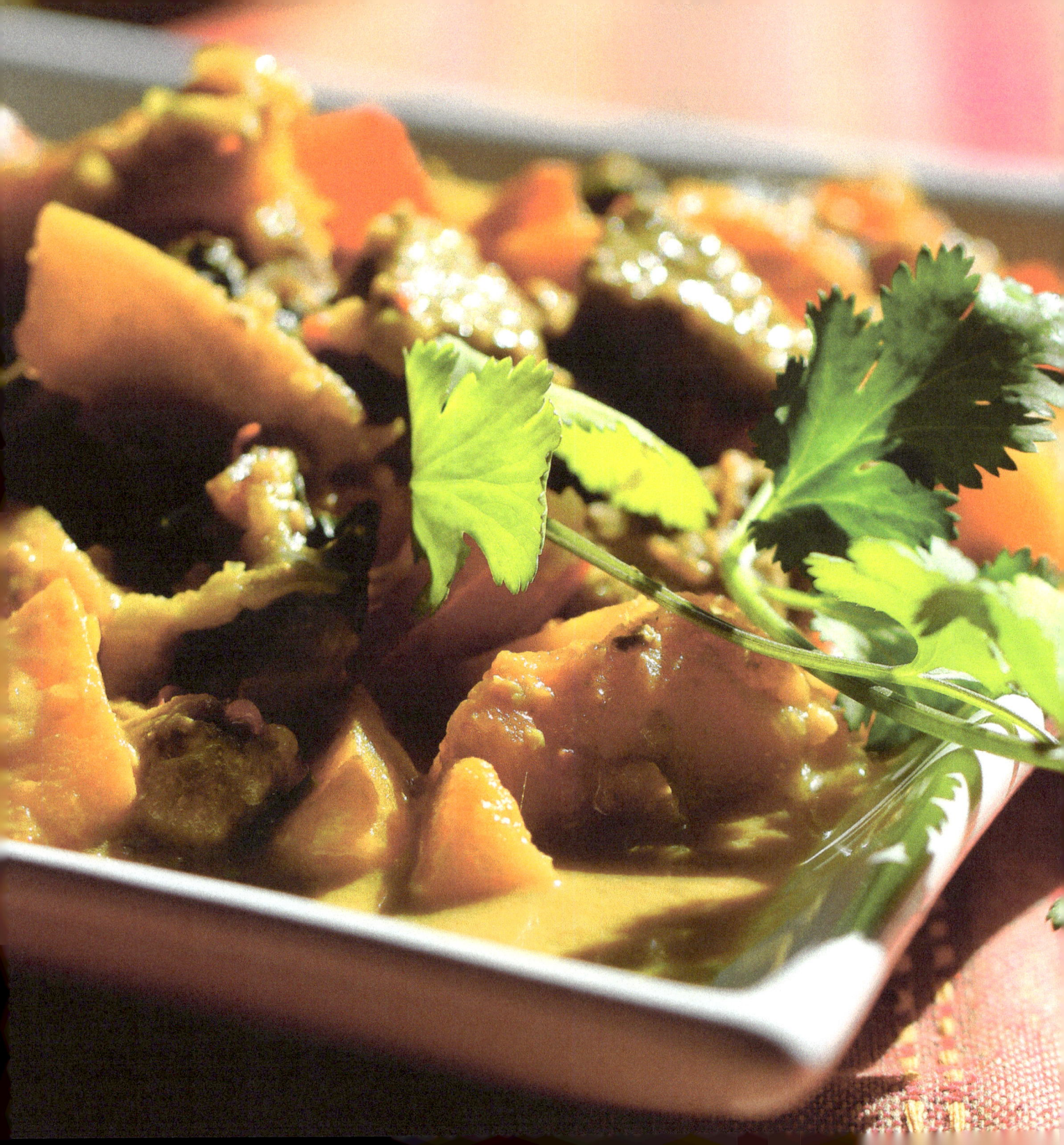

Chicken or lamb curry

Ingredients: 2 serves

500 g of diced chicken breast or lamb
1 onion diced
2 cloves garlic
2 teaspoons black mustard seeds
1-2 red chilli's (green if you do not like it hot)
2 teaspoons ginger sliced finely
2 teaspoons turmeric
2 teaspoons cumin

2 teaspoons coriander seeds
4 lime leaves
1-2 cups coconut cream or milk
1 teaspoon coconut oil
2 cups spinach
1/2 red capsicum sliced
2 cups of diced pumpkin
Juice of one lemon

Method:

Place chopped chilli, ginger, mustard and coriander seeds, turmeric, cumin, cracked pepper into a bowl and add a little coconut cream and make into a thin paste. Heat pan on low – medium heat and add coconut oil, onion and garlic stirring frequently until onions are brown then add spice paste and stir around for 2 minutes. This will release the aromas of the spices.

Then add meat to the pan, lime leaves and bring to a simmer, cover pot with a lid and simmer on low heat for 30 minutes or until meat is tender, stirring occasionally to make sure the meat is not sticking to the base of the pot. Then add pumpkin, red capsicum and spinach along with the remaining coconut cream/milk, lemon juice and a little water if required. Leave uncovered and simmer for 10-15 minutes until sauce reduces and pumpkin is soft. Serve and garnish with fresh coriander.

Homemade pizza

Ingredients: 2-4 serves

Toppings options:

Tomatoes sliced

Sundried tomatoes

Capsicum sliced

Fresh pineapple diced

Onion sliced

Eggplant diced

Cabbage sliced (optional)

Mushrooms sliced

Method:

Pre heat oven to 180 degree Celsius

To prepare base; grate cauliflower or shred in food processor, place in a glass bowl and add almond meal, flax seeds, garlic, bi-carb soda, nutritional yeast, herds and salt and pepper mix well finally add (egg optional), coconut oil and mix well. Then place mixture on baking paper on baking tray and roll out to desired thickness. Bake in the oven for 20-25 minutes until brown. While base is cooking slice up all toppings and have ready. Remove base from oven and (cover base with my home made tomato sauce optional) then add all fresh toppings of your choice. Garnish, with a sprinkle of nutritional yeast for extra flavour. Pour creamy sauce over the pizza and serve.

Place in the oven and cook for a further 10-15 minutes until toppings are hot.

High protein toppings options:

Add chicken or favourite seafood.

Creamy topping

½ cup of activated cashews

(soak cahews in warm water for 2 hours)

enough water to just cover cashews

a sprinkle of chilli powder

1 teaspoon of nutritional yeast

salt & pepper to taste

Method:

blend until creamy and pour over pizza

Pizza base

Base:

3 cups of grated cauliflower

1 ½ cups almond meal

½ cup flax seeds

1 dessertspoon of bi-carb soda (optional)

1 clove of crushed garlic

2 dessertspoons of coconut oil

2 teaspoons nutritional yeast

1 dessertspoon oregano ground dried

1 dessertspoon basil ground dried

One egg (for vegan leave out)

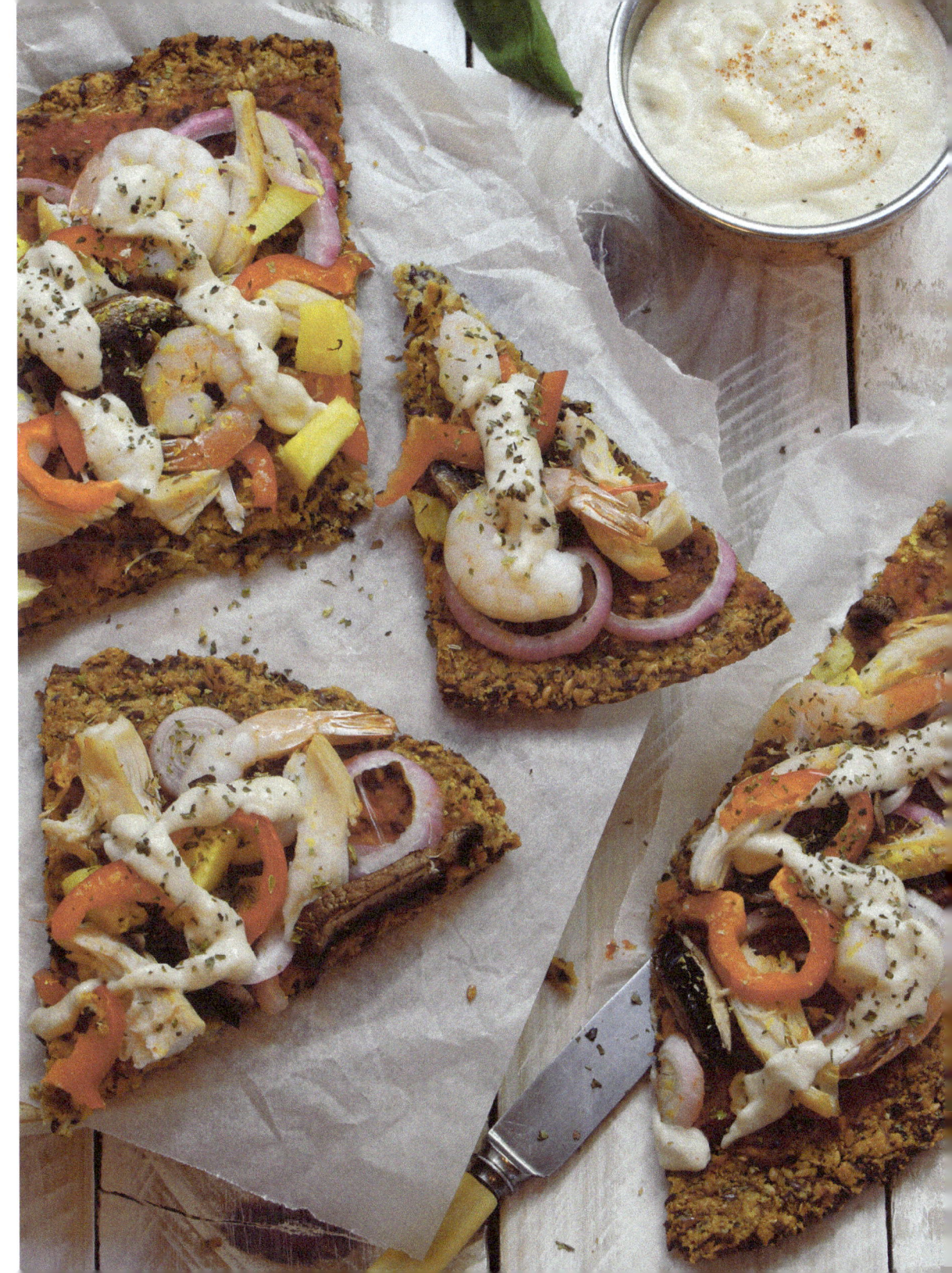

Ground beef burgers

Ingredients: 2-4 serves

400 grams of fresh ground beef

1 onion diced

1 clove of garlic

Sprinkle of nutritional yeast

1 egg

Fresh mint leaves

Pink mineral salt

Cracked black pepper

1 teaspoon of chilli powder (optional)

3 tablespoons homemade tomato sauce

Coconut flour for coating

Chia seeds for coating

Salad (baby spinach leaves, tomato, cucumber, mushroom, grated carrot & beetroot)

Homemade tomato sauce if desired

Method:

Place all ingredients into a glass bowl except the coconut flour and chia seeds and mix well. Place chia seeds and coconut flour into another small bowl and mix. Take a small amount of meat mixture and roll into a ball and roll into coconut flour and chia seed mixture and flatten out onto a plate. Repeat this until you have used all the meat mixture. Place a pan on low – medium heat with a little coconut oil once the pan is hot place the burgers in and cook until brown on both sides.

Serve on baby spinach leaves or mushroom topped with tomato, cucumber, carrot and beetroot or any other salad toppings of your choice. Finally add a little homemade tomato sauce optional.

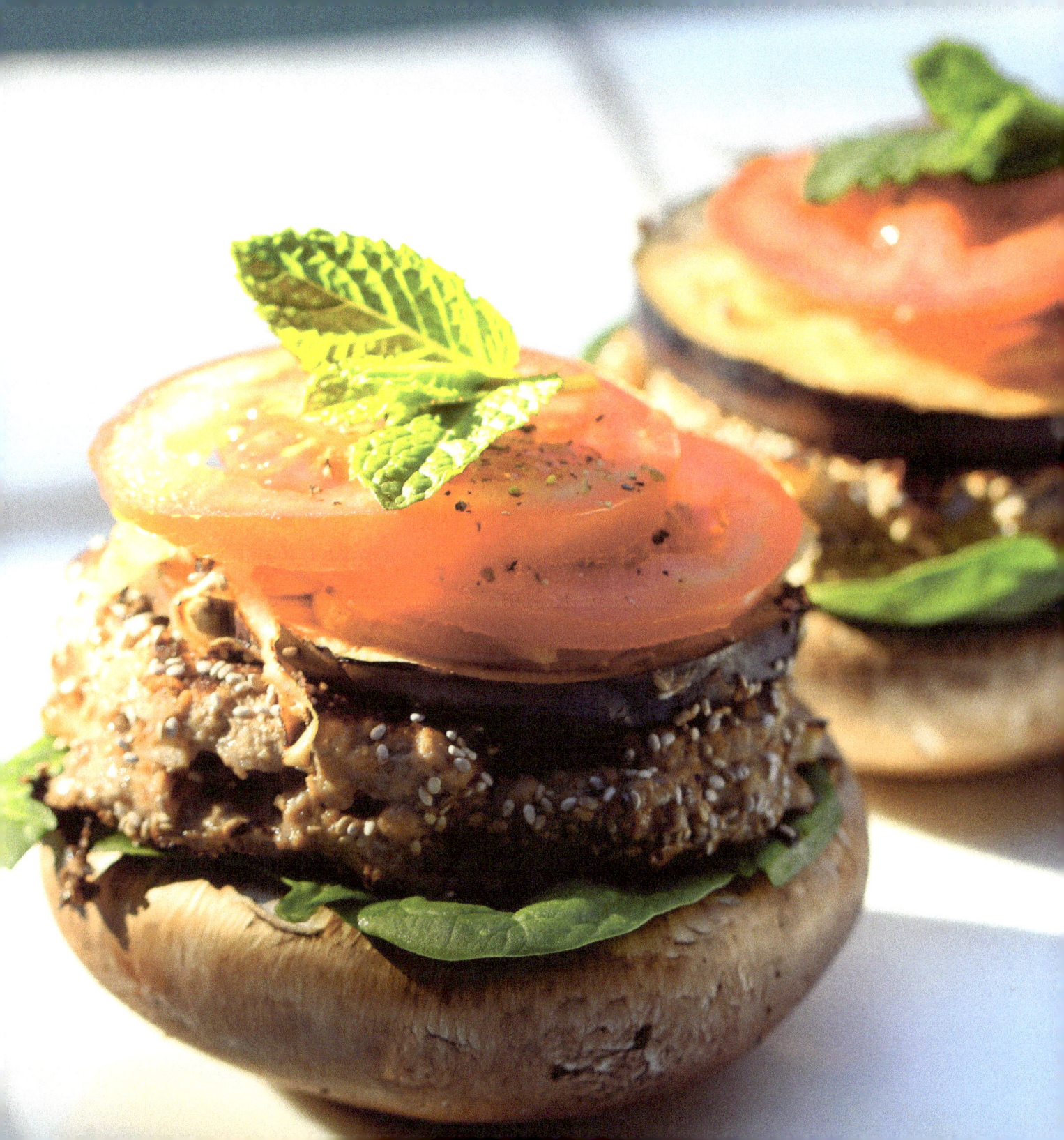

Sauté chicken kebabs

Ingredients: 2-4 serves

400-500 g of skinless chicken cubed

8 skewers

Sauté sauce (under salad dressings section)

Baby spinach leaves

4 radishes

1 lemon

Olive oil to dress salad

Pine nuts

Chia seeds or sesame seeds

Method:

Prepare the sauté sauce. Place cubed chicken onto skewers and baste with sauté sauce, then sprinkle with sesame seeds or chia seeds. Place on BBQ or under grill and cook through. Serve with salad dressed with lemon juice and olive oil. Sauté sauce can be added as dressing to salad if desired.

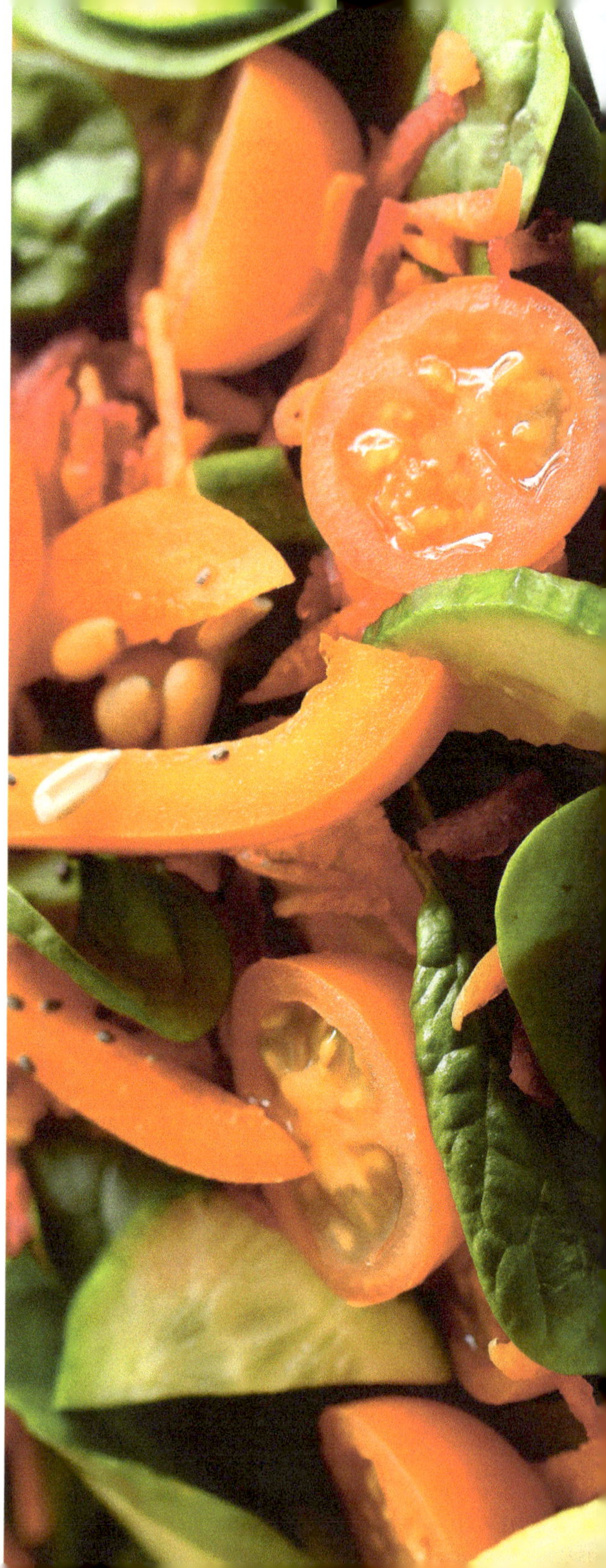

Spicy chicken kebabs

Ingredients: 2-4 serves

200-400 grams of diced chicken breast

8 green prawns

1 red & green capsicum

1 egg plant

1 onion large

Fresh pineapple

8 skewers for kebabs

1 lemon cut into wedges

Basting sauce:

1 tomato

1 clove of garlic

Cumin powder

Cinnamon powder

Chilli powder

Coconut oil

Salad:

Baby spinach leaves or rocket

2 radishes

Red & green capsicum sliced

Lemon juice and olive oil

Pine nuts

Method:

Have vegetables and pineapple chopped up into evenly sized pieces and place on skewers with chicken pieces and prawns. Mix cumin, chilli and cinnamon powder together with crushed garlic and coconut oil and blended tomato and coat the chicken and prawns on the skewers. Then place on medium heat gill and cook turning as required until cooked through. Serve with mixed salad.

Salad baby spinach leaves, sliced radishes, sliced red & green capsicum, pine nuts. Squeeze lemon juice and drizzle a little olive oil over salad as dressing.

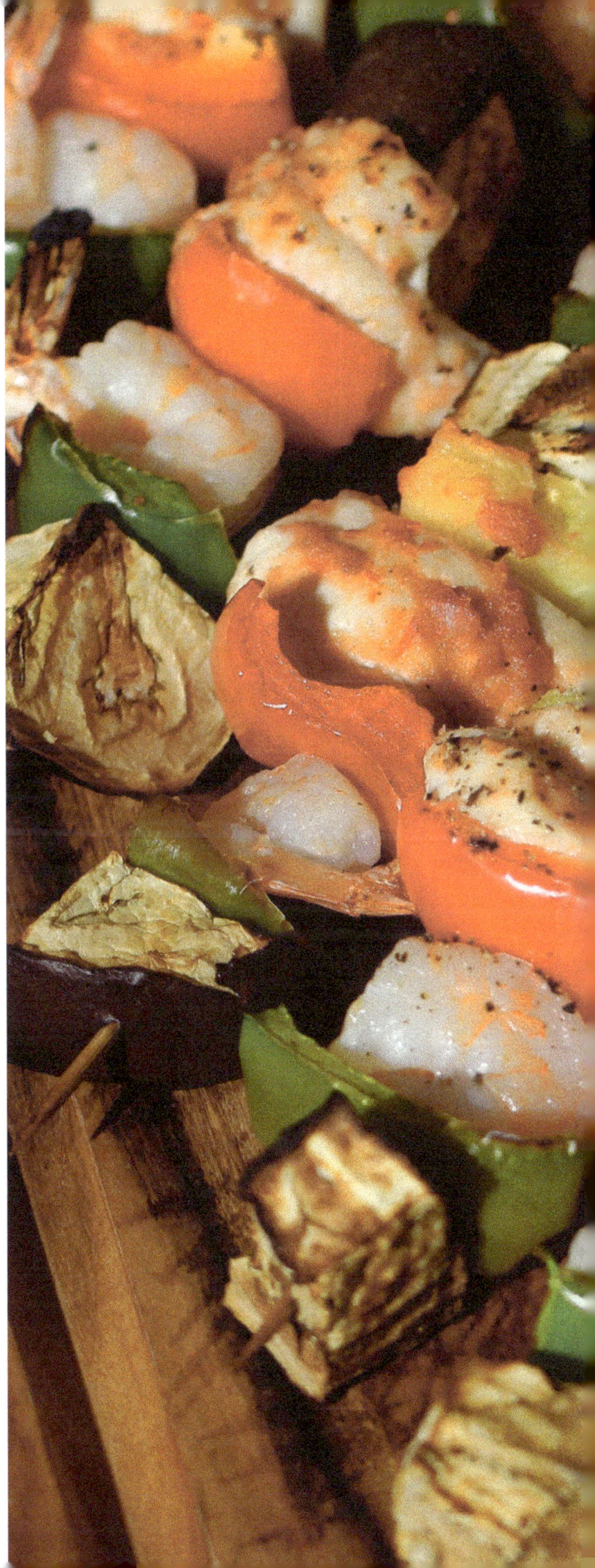

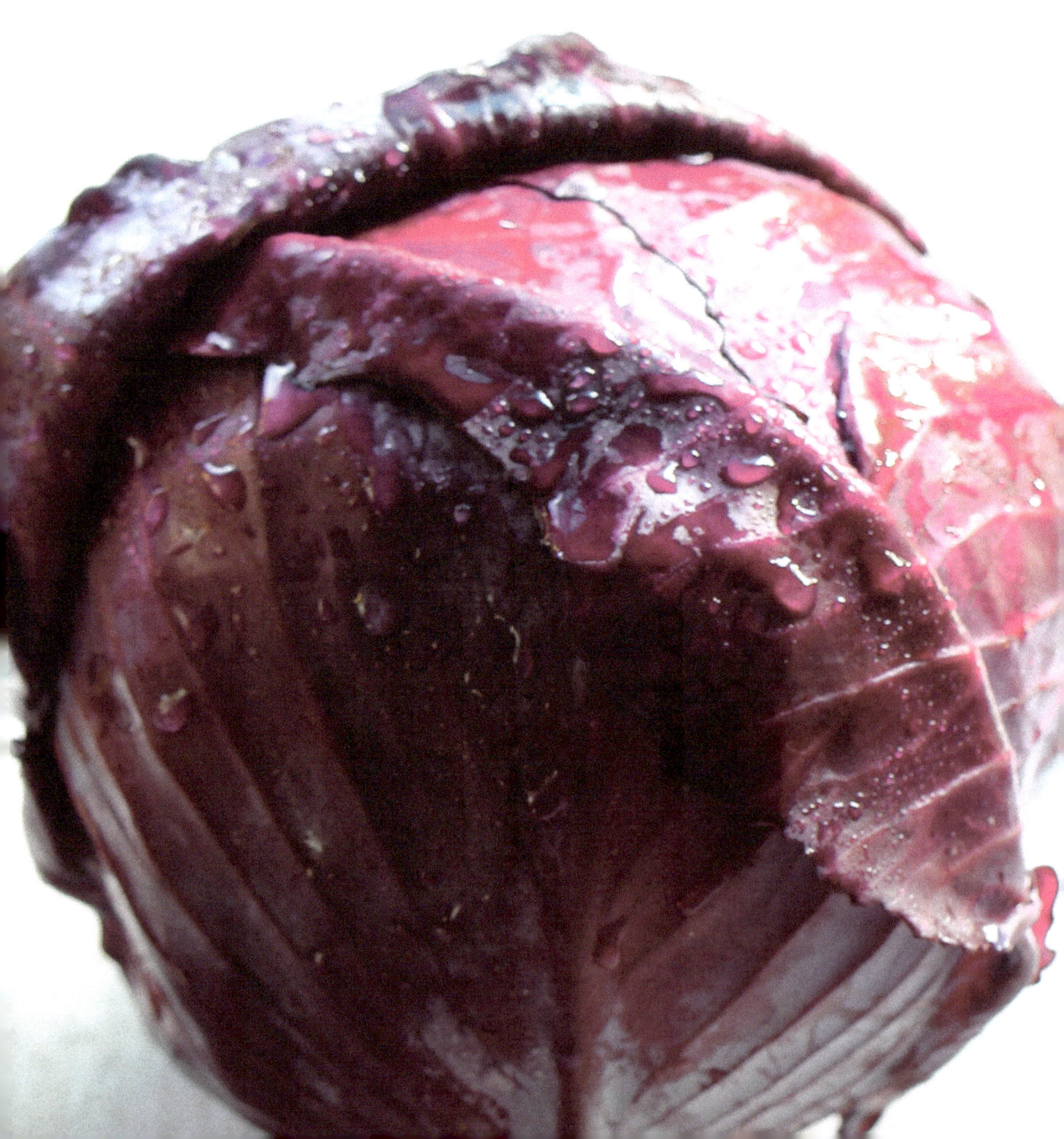

Beef cabbage rolls

Ingredients: 2-4 serves

400-500 ground beef Steak
8 cabbage leaves
1 egg
1 clove crushed garlic
1 onion
3-4 mushrooms
½ cup grated zucchini
½ diced red capsicum

½ cup grated carrot
1 teaspoon cumin powder
1 teaspoon chilli diced or powder
Sprinkle of nutritional yeast
Fresh dill to serve
Pink mineral salt & cracked black pepper to taste
Sesame seed oil
Tooth picks or string

Topped with homemade tomato sauce

Method:

Place oven on 180 degree Celsius.
Wash cabbage leaves and place in a pot of boiling salted water for 2-4 minutes until they are soft. Set aside to cool. Place onion, garlic, mushrooms and spices into pan with a little sesame seed oil and cook for several minutes, until onion is clear then add to a glass bowl with ground beef, egg, garlic, and capsicum, grated zucchini and carrot, salt and pepper.

Mix well in then place cabbage leaves out on a board and place a large spoonful of mixture into center and fold in ends. Roll up firmly to enclose filling and secure with toothpicks. Repeat with remaining cabbage leaves and mince mixture. Place remaining cabbage coarsely chopped into oven proof baking dish then add cabbage rolls on top. Pour homemade tomato sauce over. Then cover and bake for 45-50 minutes or until cooked through. Serve with fresh salad and garnish with fresh dill.

Roast lamb and mediterranean vegetables

Ingredients: 4 serves

Leg of lamb (for 4 people)
Fresh mint leaves
3 cloves garlic chopped in quarters
Pink mineral salt
Cracked black pepper
Eggplant cut into large pieces
Pumpkin 4 to 8 pieces
Beetroot 4 pieces
Red and green capsicum cut into quarters
Pine nuts
Balsamic vinegar

Method:

Preheat oven to 180 degrees Celsius. Cut slits into top of lamb and place cloves of garlic into the lamb. Place leg of lamb in baking tray with a little coconut oil into the oven. Cook for 30 minutes then turn the lamb over. Add vegetables, pumpkin, beetroot, eggplant and capsicum and cook for another 30 minutes then turn lamb and vegetables. Cook for approximately another 20 minutes, and then remove the lamb and place on a board to stand. Add balsamic vinegar and pine nuts to vegetables and return to the oven for 5 minutes turn off the oven.

Plate up; slice lamb and place with vegetables onto plates garnish with a little balsamic vinegar and pine nuts if needed.

Note: Balsamic vinegar comes in three grades. Beware of cheap imitations of balsamic vinegar. It needs to be aged and read the label on the bottle to make sure it does not have additives or artificial colouring, and thickeners. The authentic and traditional balsamic vinegar is labeled Aceto Balsamico Tradizinale and is the most expensive, aged for 12 years. Then there is the Condimento grade balsamic vinegar is usually a combination of the traditionally made product and the mass produced vinegar has grape juice added only, this is ok to use. The third is a cheap commercial grade with additives and colourings added avoid these.

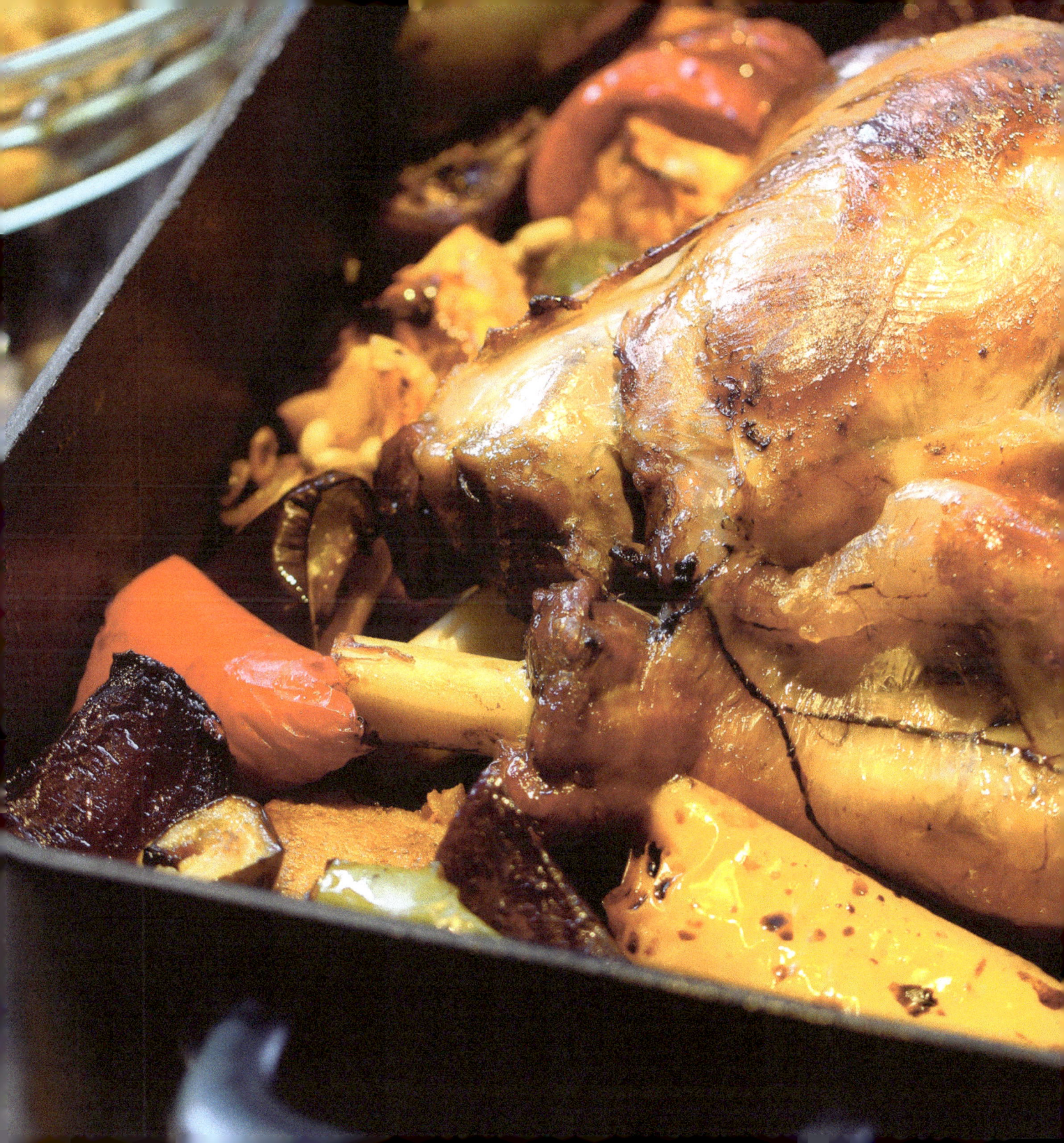

Vegetable spinach lasagna

Ingredients: 4-6 serves

- 500 g mince beef
- 2 cups of homemade tomato sauce
- 4 mushrooms
- 2 cups spinach
- 2 cups pumpkin
- 1 cup cashews (activated optional)
- Sprinkle of nutritional yeast
- 1 eggplant
- 1 clove garlic
- 1 onion
- 1 cup of shredded Cabbage
- Pinch of pink mineral salt
- Cracked black pepper to taste

Method:

Preheat oven to 180 degrees Celsius.

Place diced onion and crushed garlic into a saucepan and sauté. Then add mince beef and stir until brown, adding 1 cup of homemade tomato sauce, pepper and salt and simmer for 10 minutes. While meat sauce is cooking thinly slice eggplant and pumpkin. Place eggplant into a baking dish as bottom layer then add pumpkin on top followed by spinach. Layer, meat sauce, then cabbage, mushrooms. Repeat this layering with the eggplant, pumpkin and meat sauce.

Take the cup of cashews with ½ cup of water and blend until creamy add water as required to create a creamy consistency. Blend for approximately 20 seconds. Spread over the top of the meat mixture and bake for 40 minutes or until cooked.

Serve topped with more tomato sauce and fresh dill or basil.

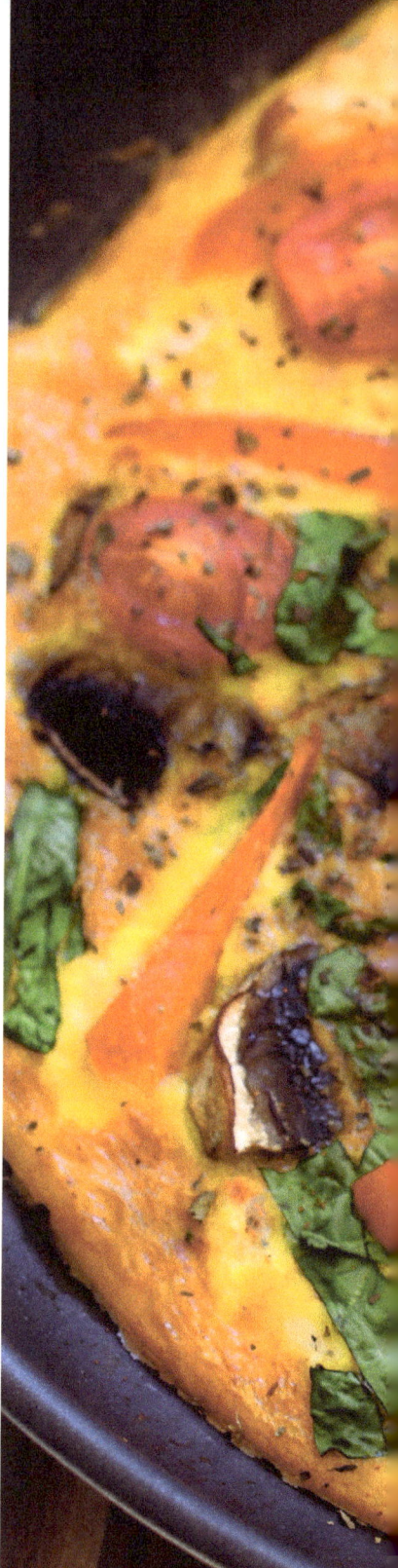

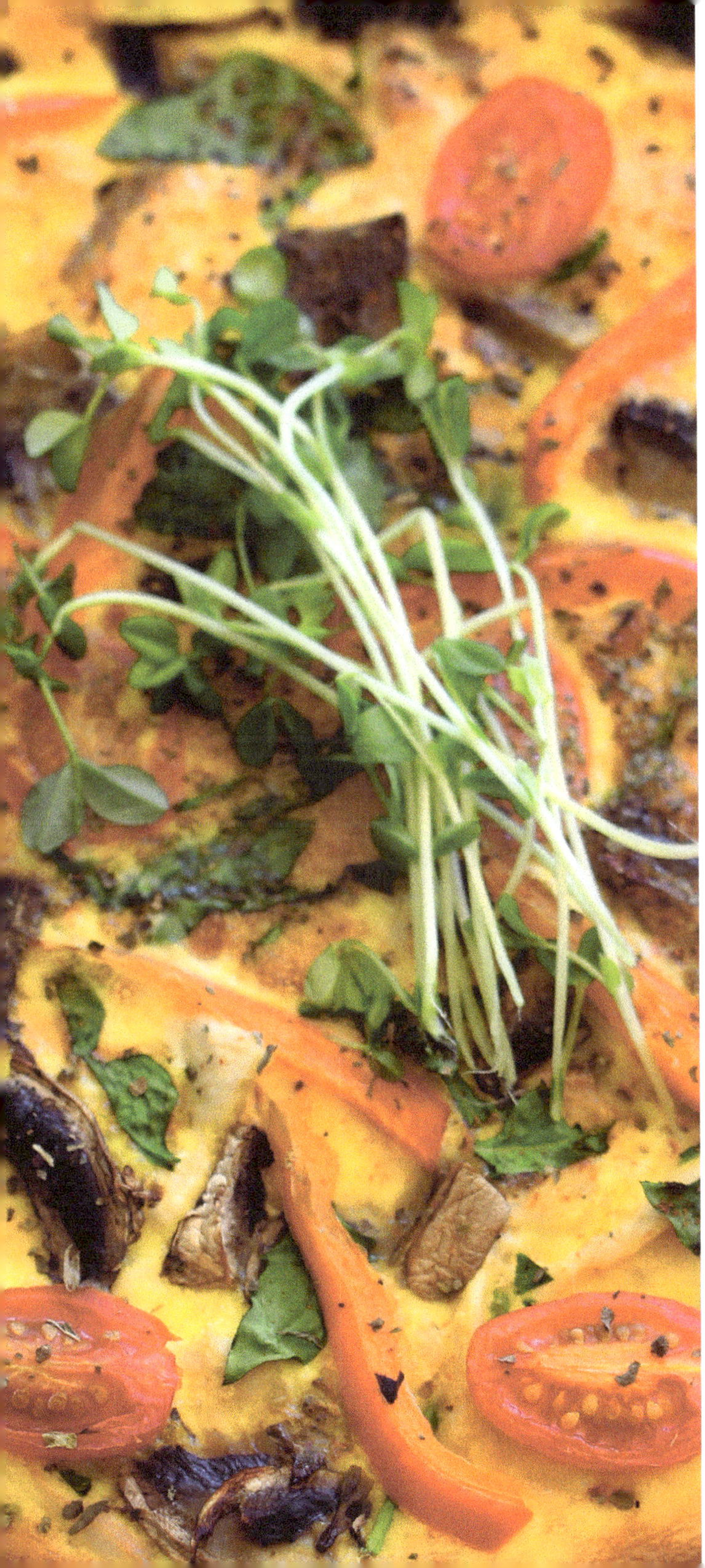

Mushroom and tomato frittata

Ingredients: 2-4 serves

4-5 eggs

½ onion or 1 spring onion

3 mushrooms

1 cup of spinach

1 tomato or 6 cherry tomatoes

½ red capsicum

1 teaspoon coconut oil

1 sprinkle of basil ground

½ a chilli diced or sprinkle of chilli powder

Pink mineral salt & cracked pepper to taste

Sprinkle of nutritional yeast

Method:

Place a pan on low to medium heat add coconut oil and sliced onion and spices cook until onion is clear. Then whisk eggs together in a small bowl and pour mixture into pan, adding sliced mushrooms, capsicum, tomato, spinach, basil, salt, pepper and nutritional yeast cook until the eggs are almost set. Then place pan under a grill until top is cooked. Serve with fresh salad.

Add: sliced cooked Atlantic salmon or shredded cooked chicken for high protein option

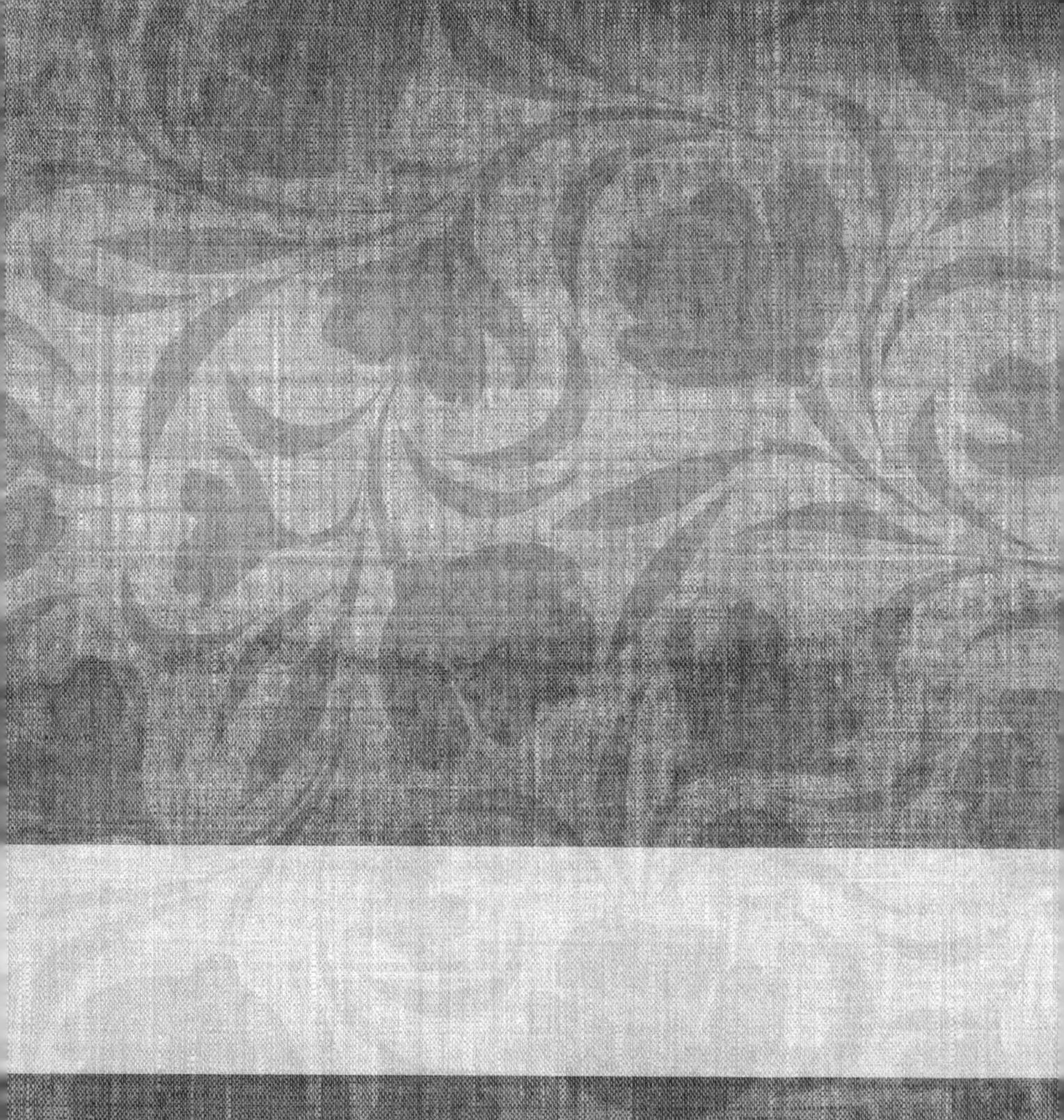

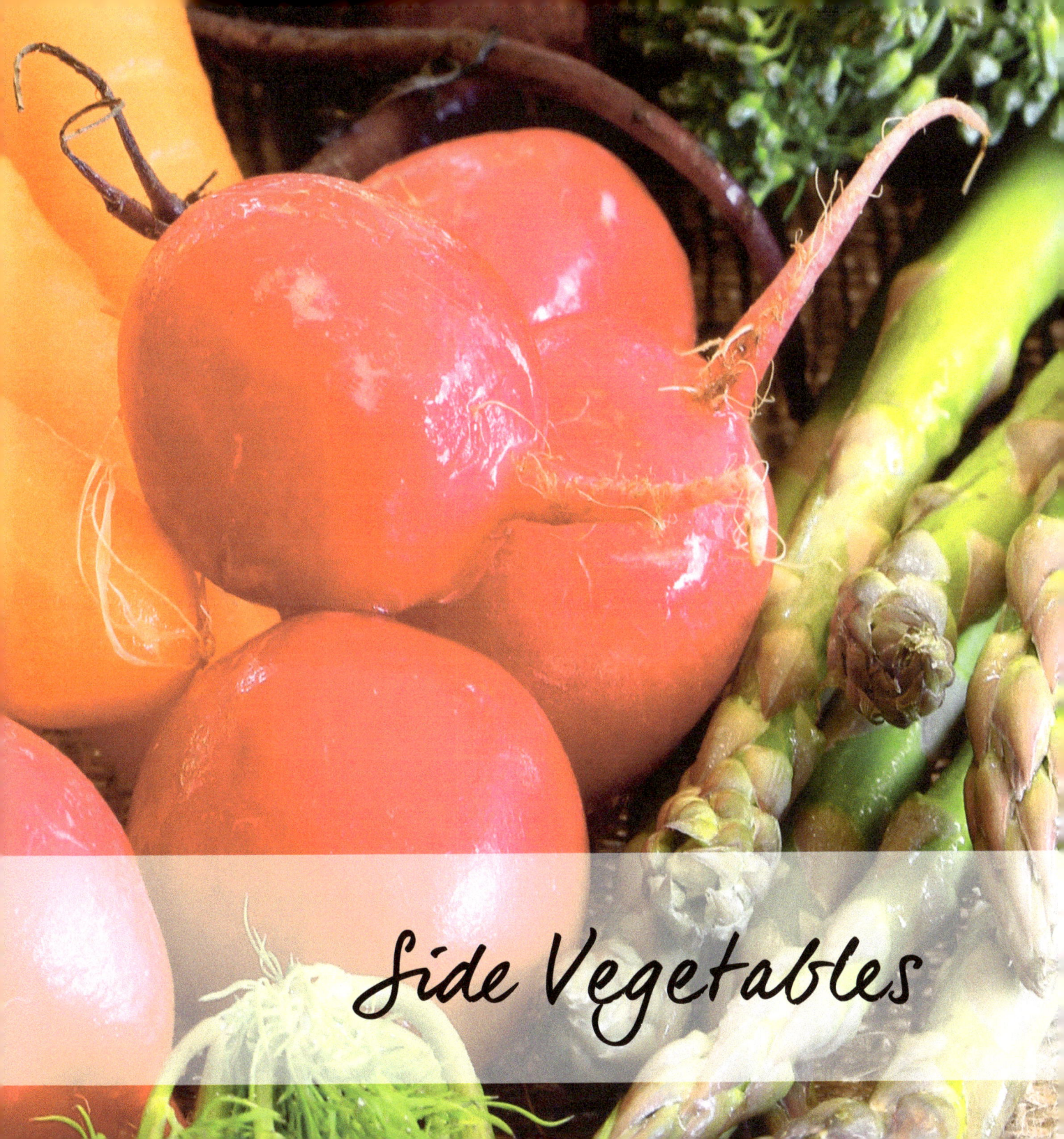
Side Vegetables

Baked sweet potato wedges

Ingredients: 2-4 serves

8-12 pieces of sweet potatoes (depends on the size)
Cracked black pepper, to taste
Pink mineral salt (optional)
1 tablespoon of coconut oil
1 clove of crushed garlic
1 teaspoon of grated ginger
1 teaspoon of paprika or chilli ground
2 teaspoons of cumin ground
2 teaspoons of cinnamon ground

Method:

Preheat oven to 180 degrees Celsius. Wash and cut sweet potato into wedges. Place all other ingredients into a bowl and mix well, then baste the sweet potato wedges. Bake for 30-40 minutes or until soft in the middle. Sweet potato wedges go well with roast meat and chicken.

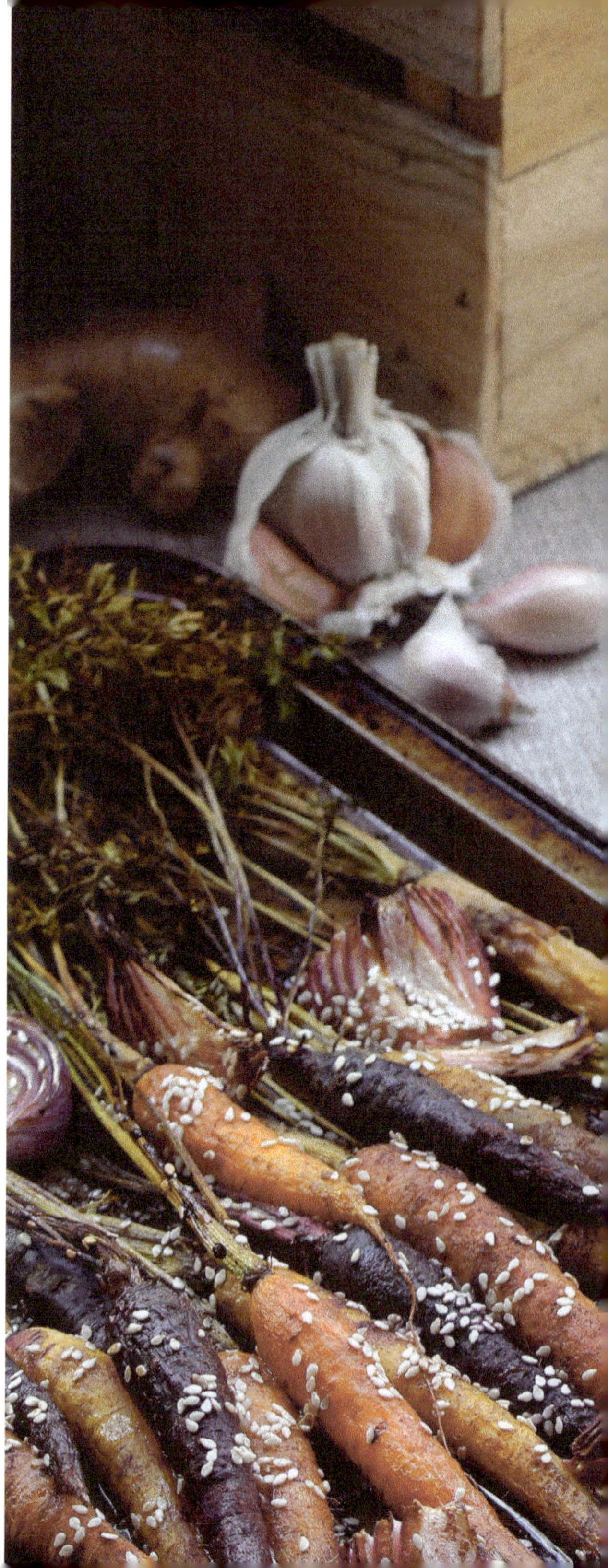

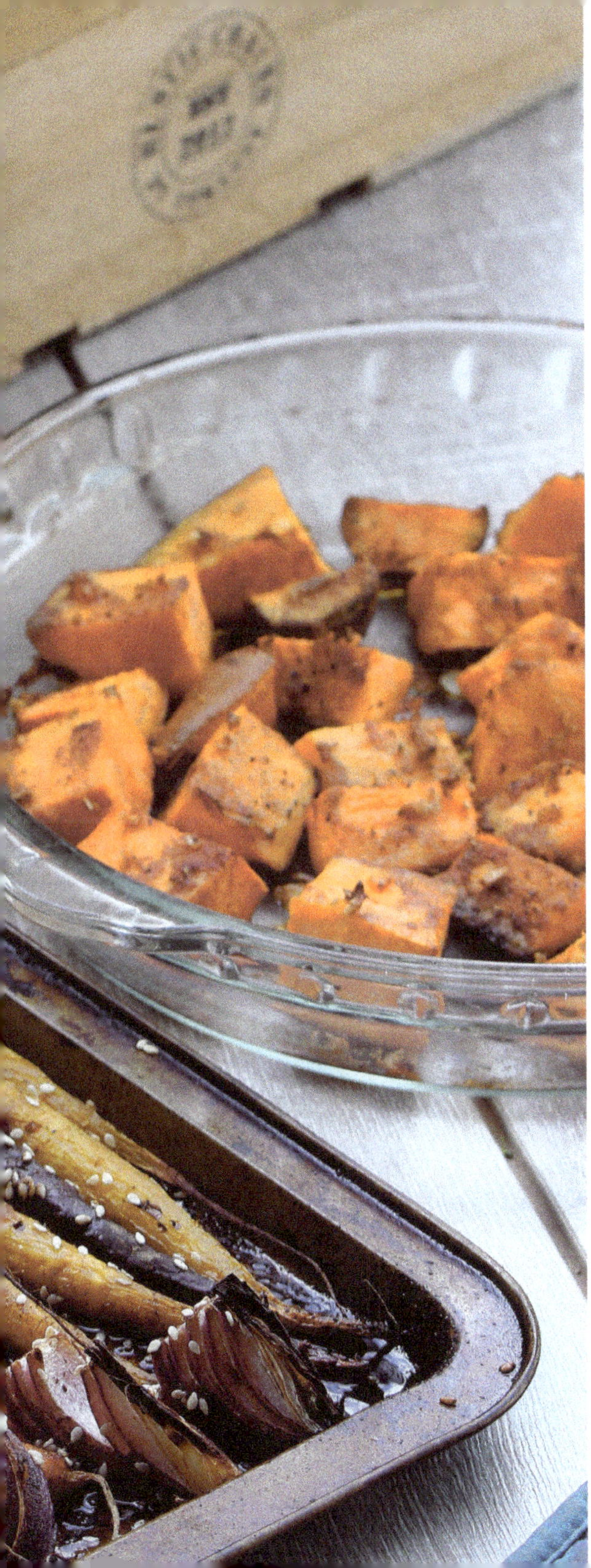

Baked carrots

Ingredients: 2-4 serves

1 bunch of baby carrots
1 medium red onion
¼ cup sesame seeds
1 dessertspoon organic honey (optional)
1 tablespoon of coconut oil
1 dessertspoon of cinnamon ground
½ cup of balsamic vinegar

Method:
Preheat oven to 180 degrees Celsius.
Place washed carrots into an oven proof dish with peeled onion cut into 8 pieces. Then place remaining ingredients into a small bowl and mix well, then pour over carrots and onions and bake for 20 minutes turning the carrots and onions if needed. Goes beautifully with roast meat or chicken.

Baked zucchini

Ingredients: 2-4 serves
4-6 zucchinis
1 red onion
1 clove of crushed garlic
Black cracked pepper to taste
½ teaspoon pink mineral salt
2 tablespoons nutritional yeast
½ cup cashews (Activated optional)
2 teaspoons of coconut oil

Method:
Preheat oven to 180 degrees Celsius.
Slice onion into rings and fry on a low heat in coconut oil until clear. Then place the onions into an oven proof dish, slice up the zucchini and layer over the onions. Then add crushed garlic salt and pepper.

Place the cashews into the blender and add nutritional yeast and blend until the mixture resembles bread crumbs. Sprinkle over the zucchini and bake for 30 minutes or until golden brown.

Steamed vegetables

Ingredients: 2-4 serves
2 cups of broccoli pieces
1 cup green beans
½ red capsicum large slices
4-6 small pieces sweet potato
1 cup of baby spinach leaves
Cracked black pepper
½ teaspoon pink mineral salt
Homemade tomato sauce (dressing)
Creamy sauté sauce (dressing)

Method:
Place sweet potato, into the steamer for four minutes then add broccoli, beans, and red capsicum for 2 minutes then turn off the heat and add baby spinach leaves. Then place in a serving bowl topped with pepper and salt, and serve. Homemade tomato sauce, creamy capsicum sauce or creamy sauté sauce can be added for extra taste (recipes in salad dressing section).

Baked mediterranean vegetables

Ingredients: 2-4 serves

2 small beetroot

4-6 pieces of pumpkin

1 onion

1 egg plant

¼ cup pine nuts

1 tablespoon of coconut oil

4-6 tablespoons of good quality Balsamic vinegar

Method:

Preheat oven to 180 degrees Celsius. Place washed and evenly sized sliced vegetables into a baking dish with a little coconut oil. Bake for 40 minutes or until soft, turning at the 20 minute mark. Then add pine nuts and balsamic vinegar and cook for a further 5 minutes. Makes a great side dish with roast meat or chicken.

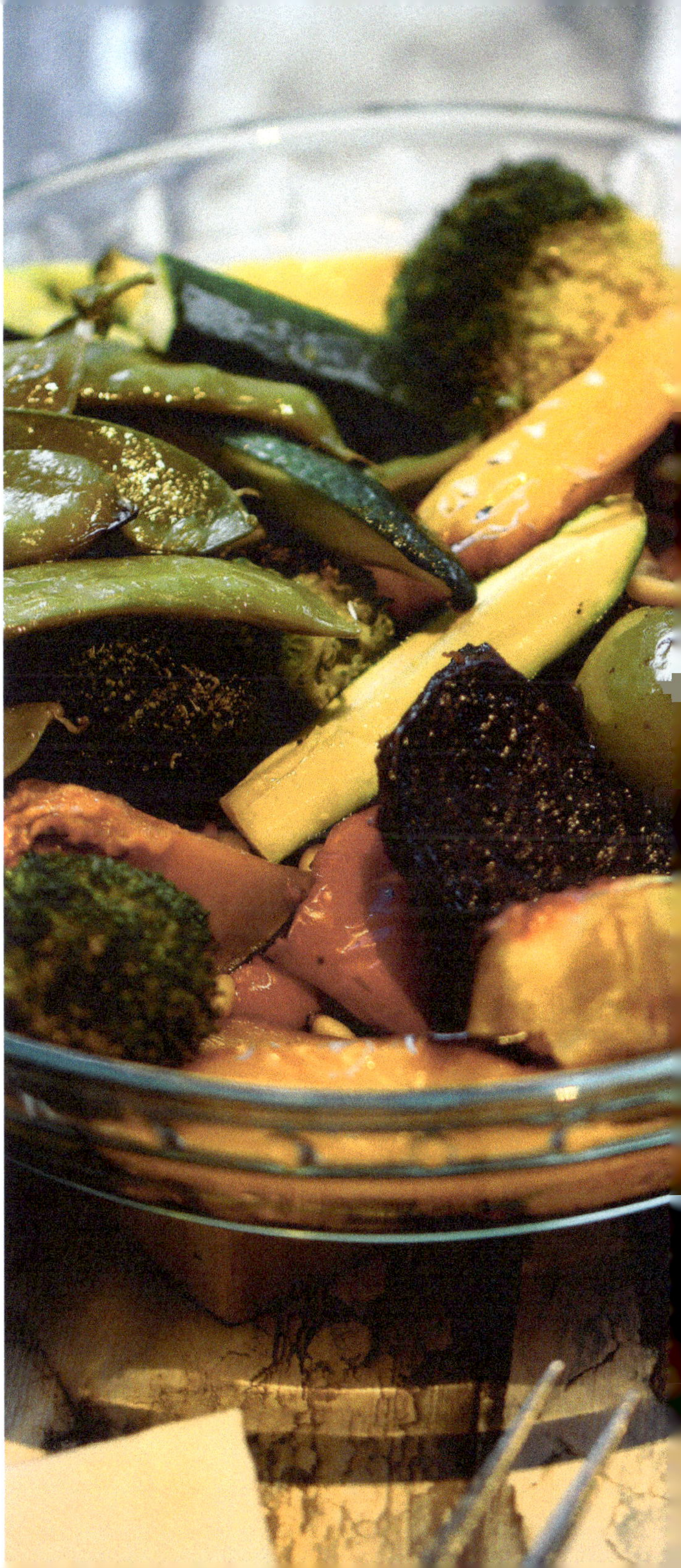

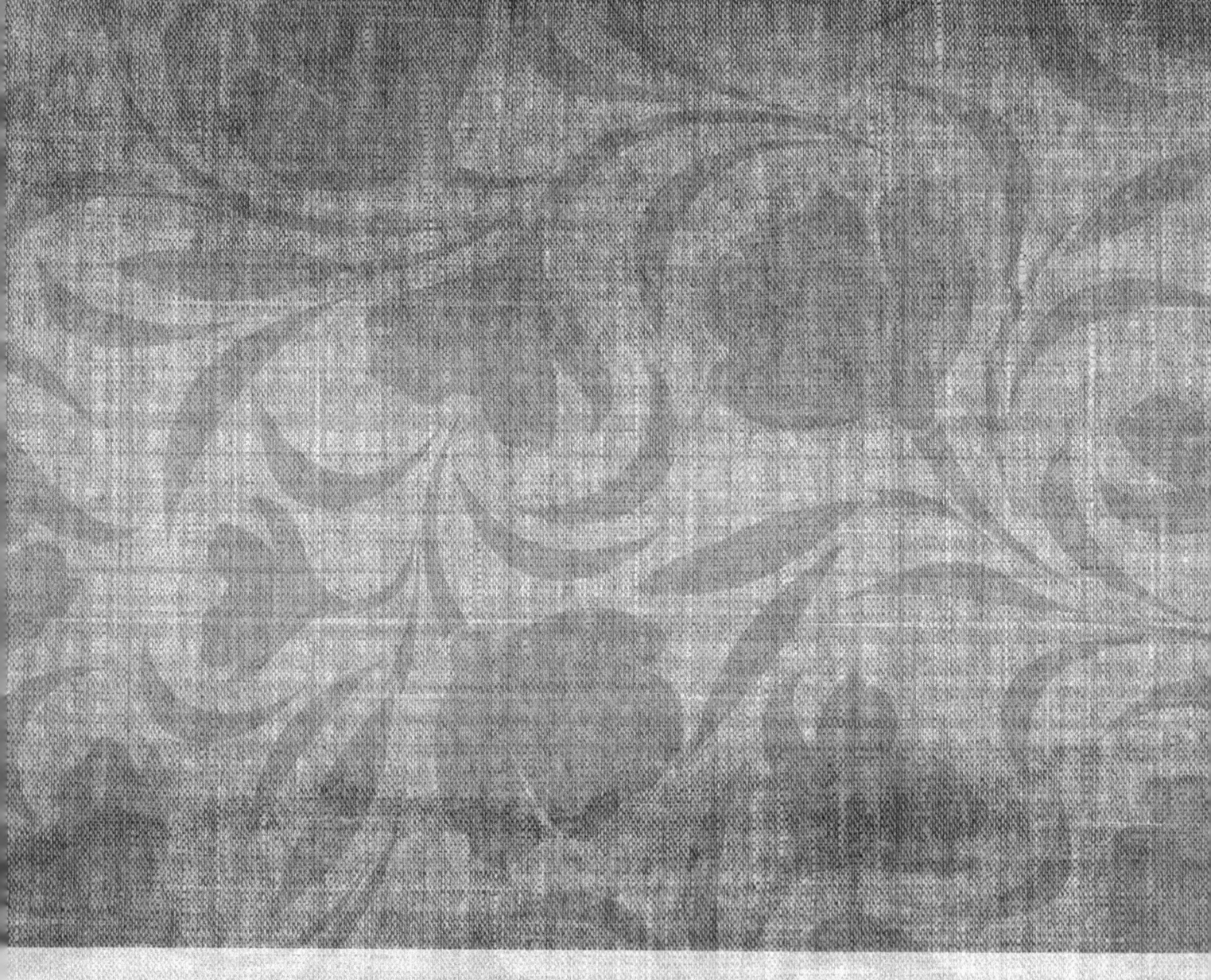

Benefits Of pumpkin, sunflower and sesame seeds

Raw pumpkin seeds or Pepitas provide a rich source of fibre which benefits digestive health. They are high in protein and minerals such as iron, potassium, phosphorus, zinc and magnesium.

Sunflower and sesame seeds are similar to pumpkin seeds, they are also a great source of health benefiting nutrients, minerals, antioxidants and vitamins.

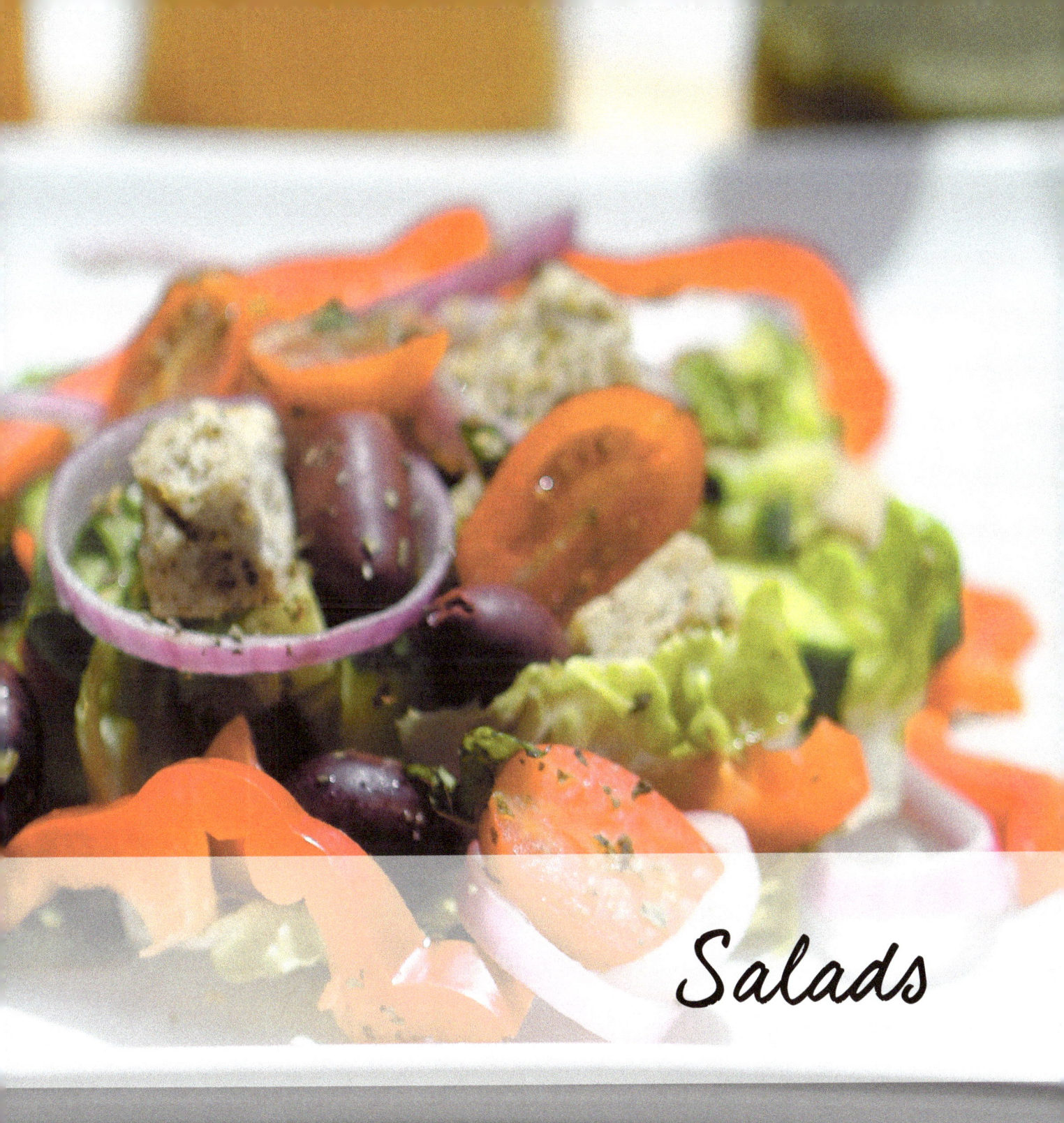

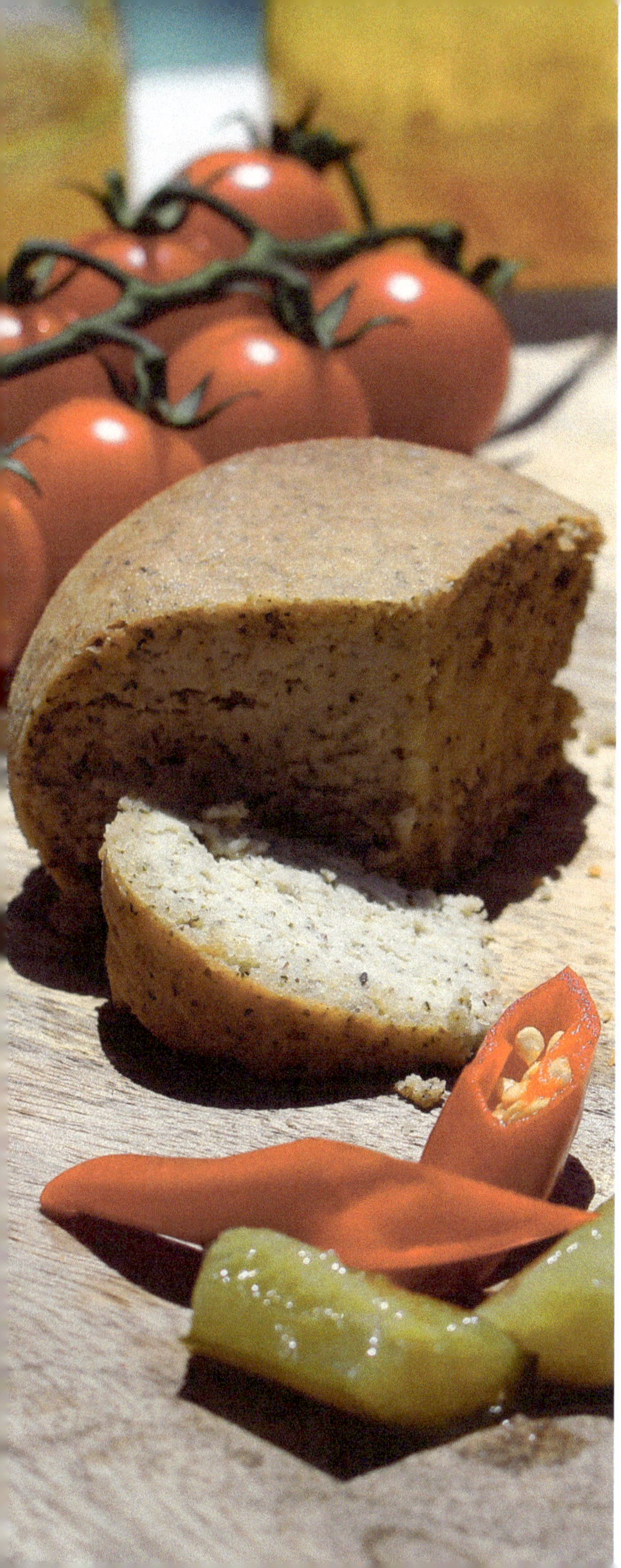

Almond feta

Ingredients:

1 cup of almond meal
½ cup of brazil nuts
¼ cup of lemon juice
1/2 cup water
3 tablespoons of olive oil
2 tablespoons of nutritional yeast
1 clove crushed garlic
1 teaspoon of pink mineral salt
Cracked pepper to taste
1 dessertspoon of dried oregano
1 dessertspoon of dried basil

Method:

Place brazil nuts into a blender and blend until a fine mixture then add all other ingredients to the blender and blend until a creamy texture. Remove an place into a cheese cloth in a colander inside a large bowl to drain in the fridge for 10 Hours. Preheat oven to 180 degrees Celsius. Remove the mixture from the cheese cloth and place in an oven proof bowl and bake for 40 minutes or until golden brown on the outside. Allow to cool then slice into cubes and serve on the greek salad.
Also ideal as a cheese alternative on crackers with tomato or served with fermented cucumbers and peppers.

Note: For another flavour option replace oregano and basil with ½ a red capsicum.

Greek salad

Ingredients: 2-4 serves

1 cup of cherry tomatoes
1 medium red onion
1 large lebanese cucumber
1 green capsicum
1 red capsicum
½ cup fresh mint
½ cup of pitted olives
2 teaspoons of dried oregano
Sprinkle of nutritional yeast
Cracked black pepper
Pink mineral salt
¼ cup extra virgin olive oil
¼ cup of apple cider vinaigrette dressing
(under salad dressing section)
Almond feta cubes
Cos lettuce (optional)

Method:

Place diced cucumber, thinly sliced onion, capsicums and cherry tomatoes sliced in half into a salad bowl, then add finely chopped mint, olives, oregano, nutritional yeast and pepper and salt. Then add the almond feta and dressings and toss gently and serve.

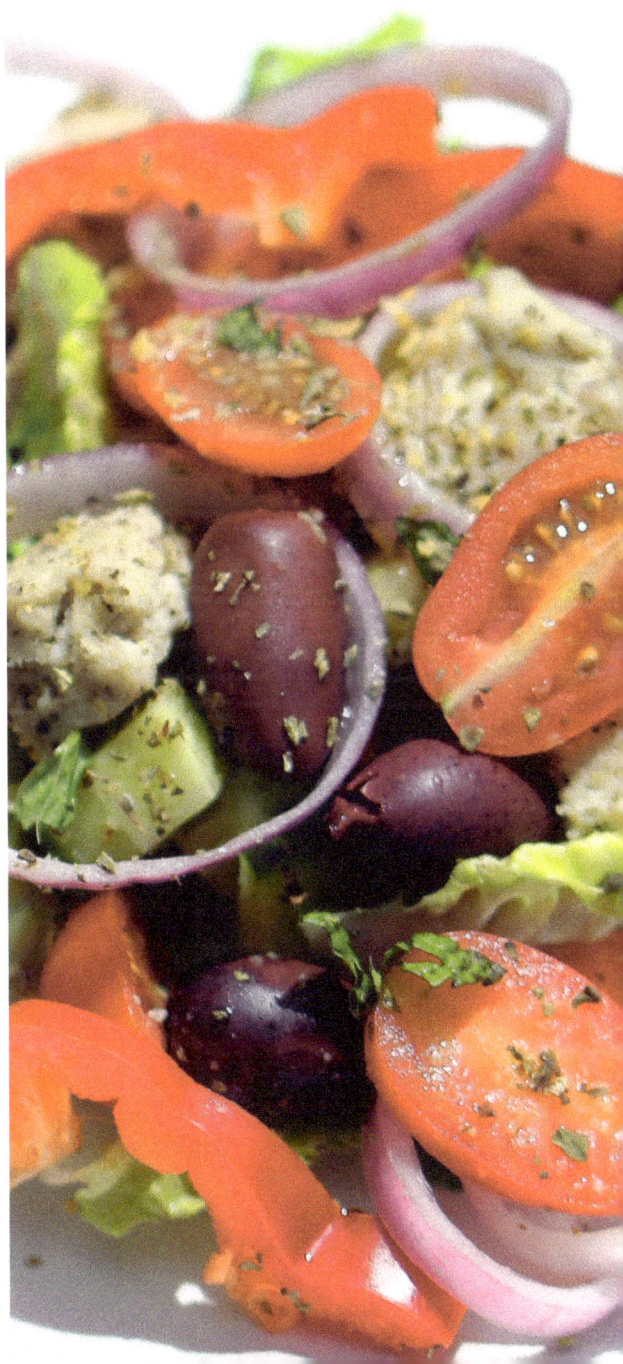

Raw beetroot & carrot salad

Ingredients: 2-4 serves
2 beetroots
1 carrot
3 radishes
2 spring onions

Method:
Grate washed beetroots and carrot or if you have a vegetable spiralizer use it for the carrot & beetroot. Then thinly slice the radish and spring onions, and dress with a little lemon juice or one of the salad dressings in the dressing section. Garnish with sunflower kernels

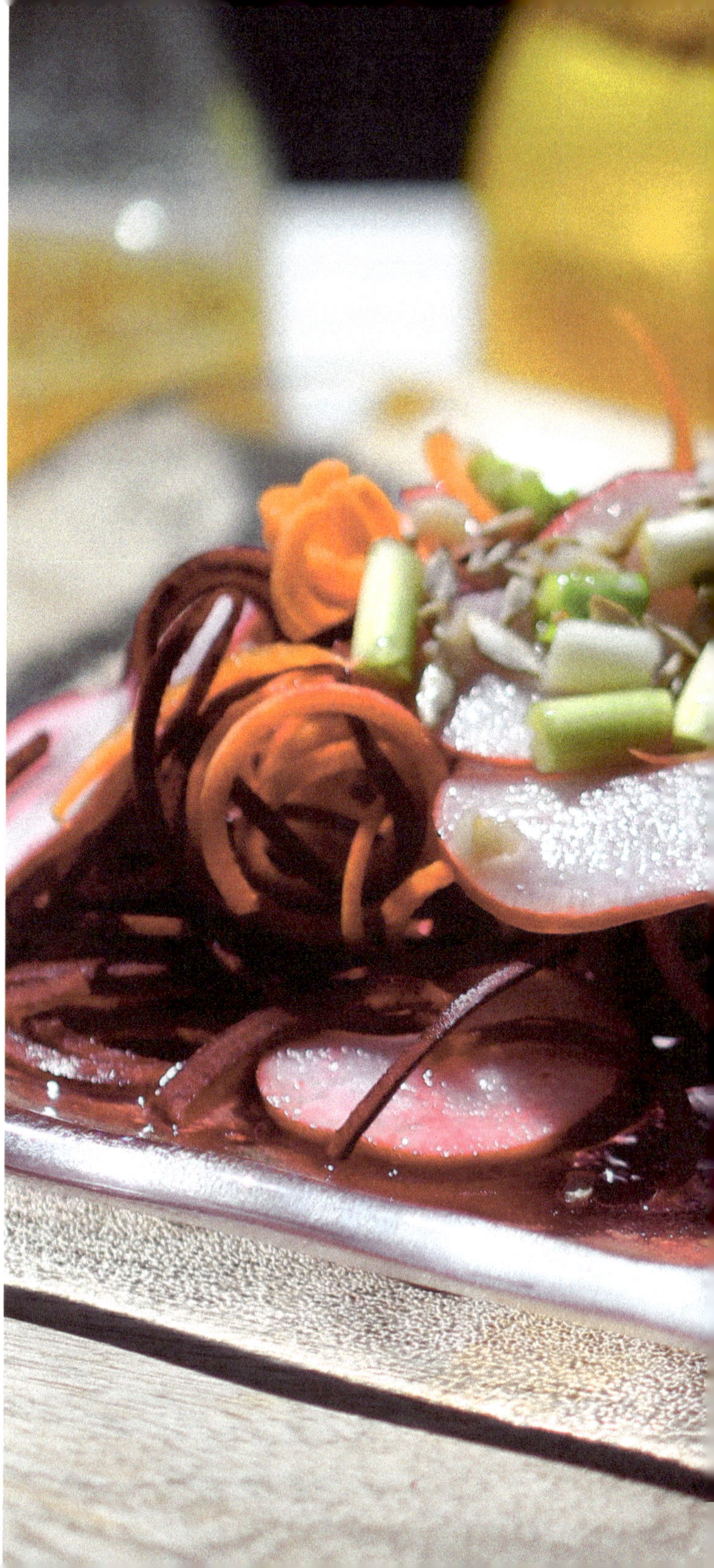

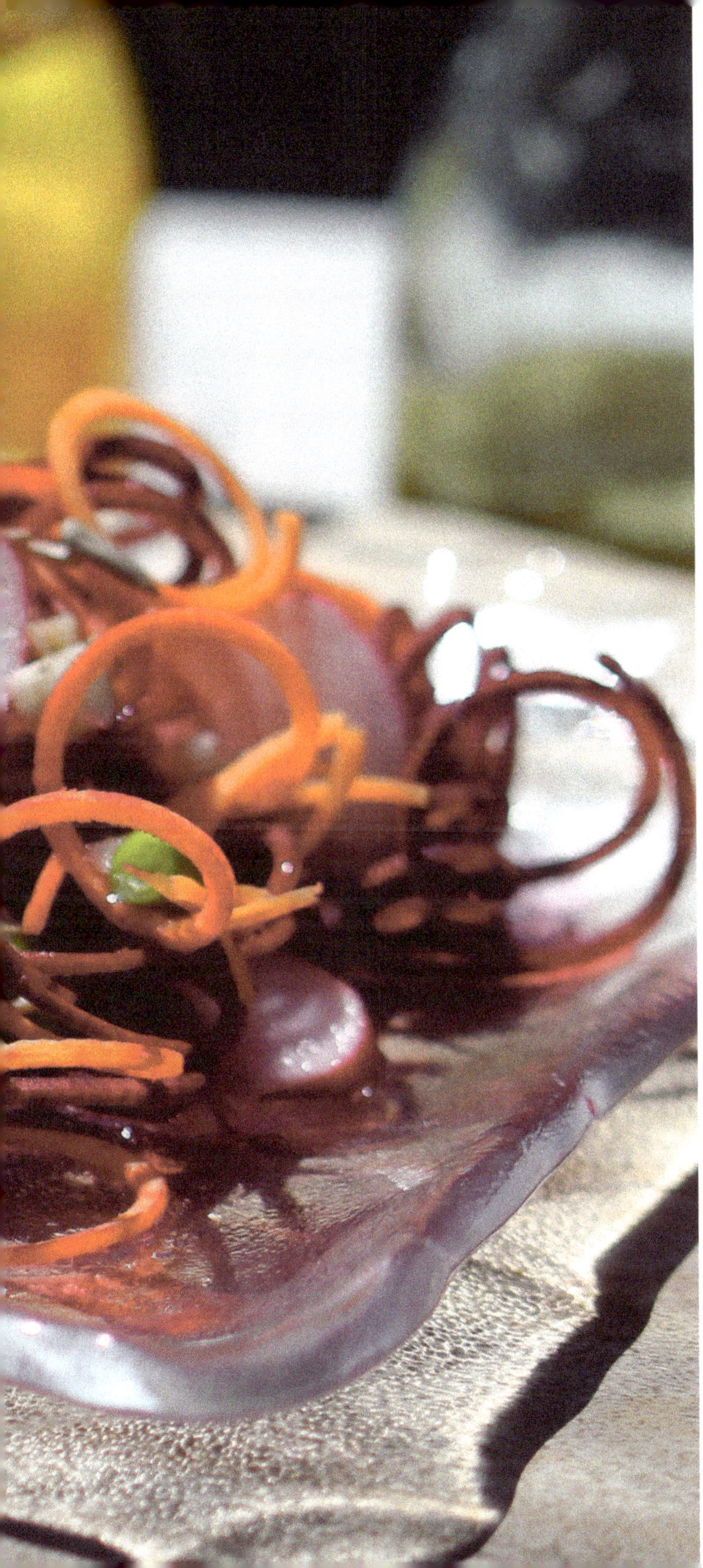

Pear apple & almond salad

Ingredients: 2-4 serves

1 bowl of mixed greens
2 pears
1 apples
½ cup of slivered almonds
6 prunes
Fresh mint garnish
½ cup of apple cider vinaigrette dressing (under salad dressing section)

Method:

Place washed mixed greens into a glass salad bowl. Then diced apple, pears and prunes and add to mixed greens. Top with slivered almonds and fresh mint and apple cider vinegar vinaigrette dressing, gently toss and serve.

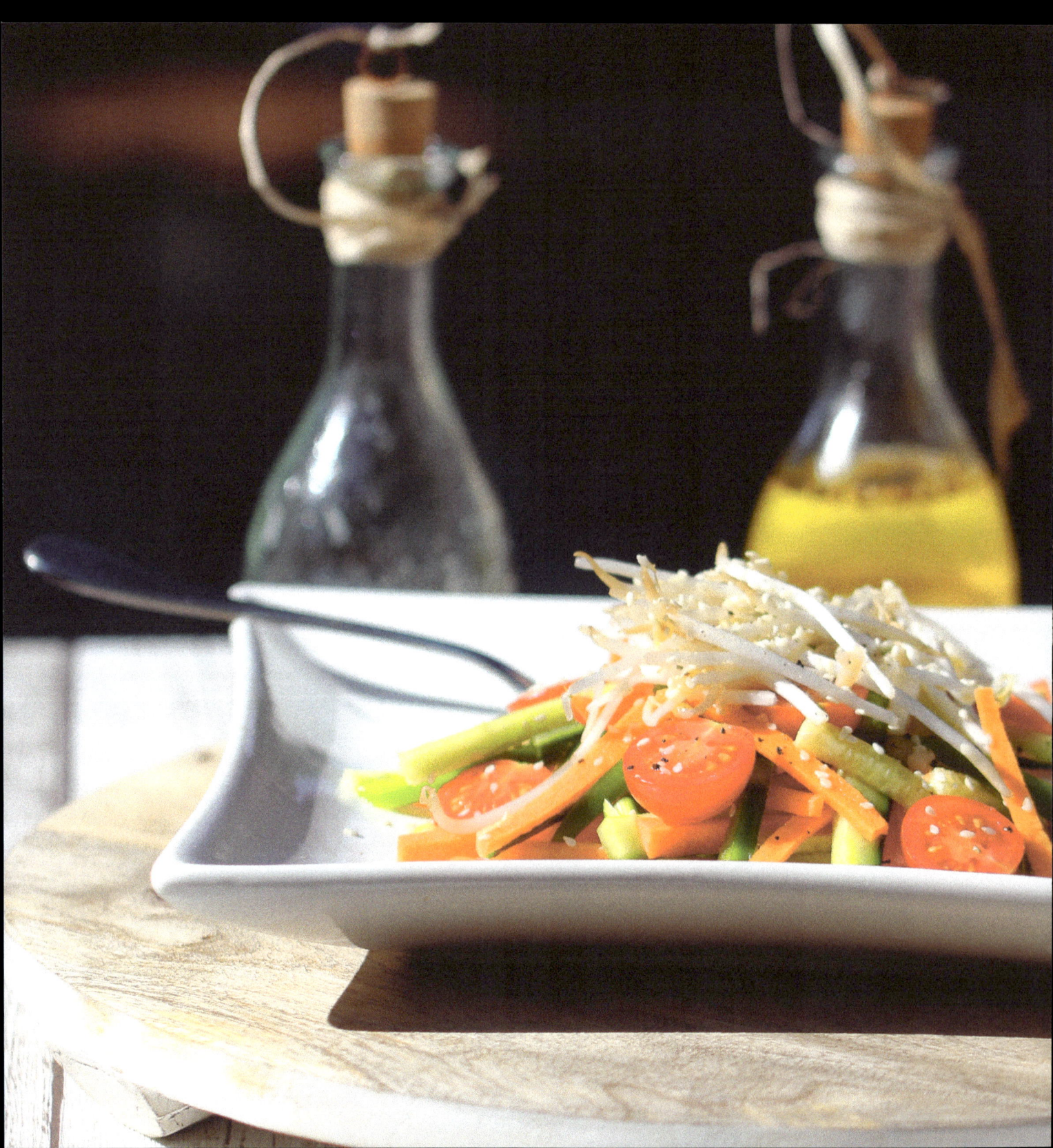

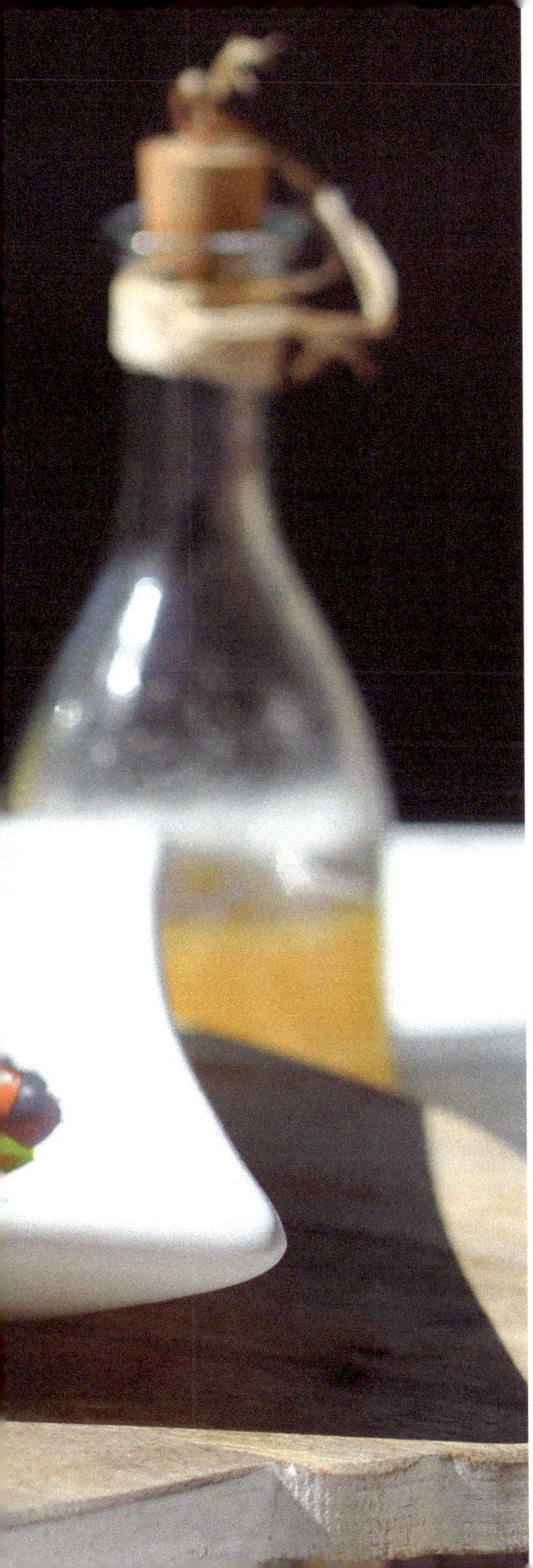

Spring salad

Ingredients: 2-4 serves

1 cucumber
1 carrot
½ red capsicum
½ green capsicum
6 cherry tomatoes
1 cup of bean sprouts
1 spring onion
1 tablespoon Sesame seeds (optional)

Method:
Cut cucumber, capsicum and carrot into matchsticks, and add to a glass bowl. Then add tomatoes sliced into halves and spring onions finely sliced to other ingredients. Then add bean sprouts and sesame seeds, and apple cider vinaigrette dressing. Gently toss and serve.

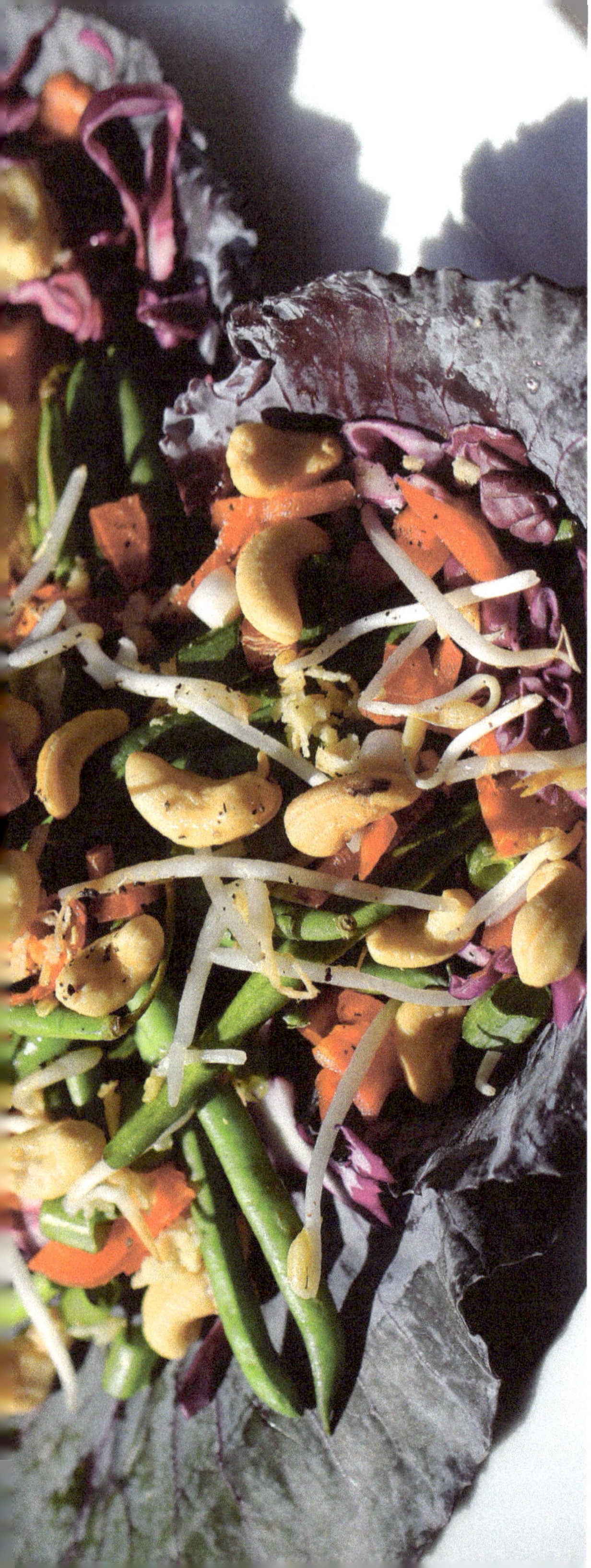

Asian salad

Ingredients: 2-4 serves

2 cups of green beans
½ cup fresh coriander
½ red cabbage
½ red capsicum
½ cup of bean sprouts
1 spring onion
¼ cup of cashew nuts
1 teaspoon of grated ginger
1 fresh chilli
2 tablespoons of lime juice
1 teaspoon of sesame seed oil (olive oil can substitute)
Black cracked pepper
Pink mineral Salt to taste

Method:

Place beans in a steamer for 2 minutes to blanche then, remove from heat and place into a glass salad bowl. Thinly slice coriander, red cabbage, red capsicum, chilli and spring onion and add to beans. Top with bean sprouts and cashews and gently mix. Place the lime juice, sesame seed oil, grated ginger, pepper & salt into a small mixing bowl stir well. Pour the salad dressing over the salad and gently toss dressing through. Refrigerate for 20 minutes allowing the beans to cool and salad dressing flavors to infuse through the salad.

Note: Cooked sliced chicken can be added to make a complete high protein meal option.

Chia mixed salad

Ingredients: 2-4 serves

1 bunch of Pak choy or Bok choy (Chinese white cabbage)
6-10 Snow peas
1 stick Celery
2 spring onions
½ green capsicum
¼ cup slivered almonds
Sprinkle sesame seeds
1 teaspoon of ginger
1 clove of crushed garlic
1 teaspoon of sesame seed oil
1 lemon (juice)
Cracked black pepper, to taste
1 chilli
1 tablespoon Chia seeds

Method:

Place chopped Pak/Bok choy, snow peas, into a pan on low with a little water and place a lid on it for 2 minutes to blanche the Choy and peas. Meanwhile slice spring onions and capsicum and set aside. Then drain and place the Pak/Bok choy and snow peas into a serving plate and top with, diagonally sliced celery, slivered almonds and sesame seeds and chia seeds. Prepare salad dressing by using a small glass bowl and adding sliced or grated ginger, lemon juice, crushed garlic and sesame seed oil, pepper and sliced chilli together and mix well. Then pour over the salad and serve.

Note: For a high protein option add cooked prawns or fish.

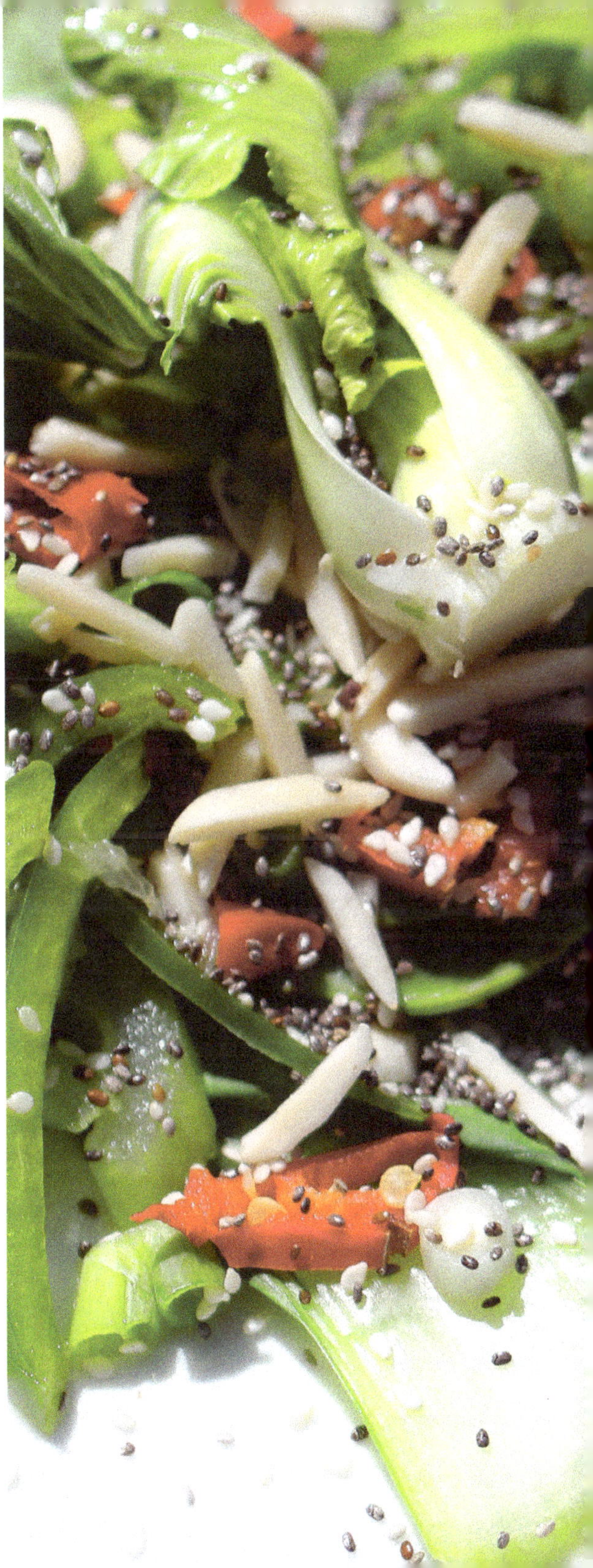

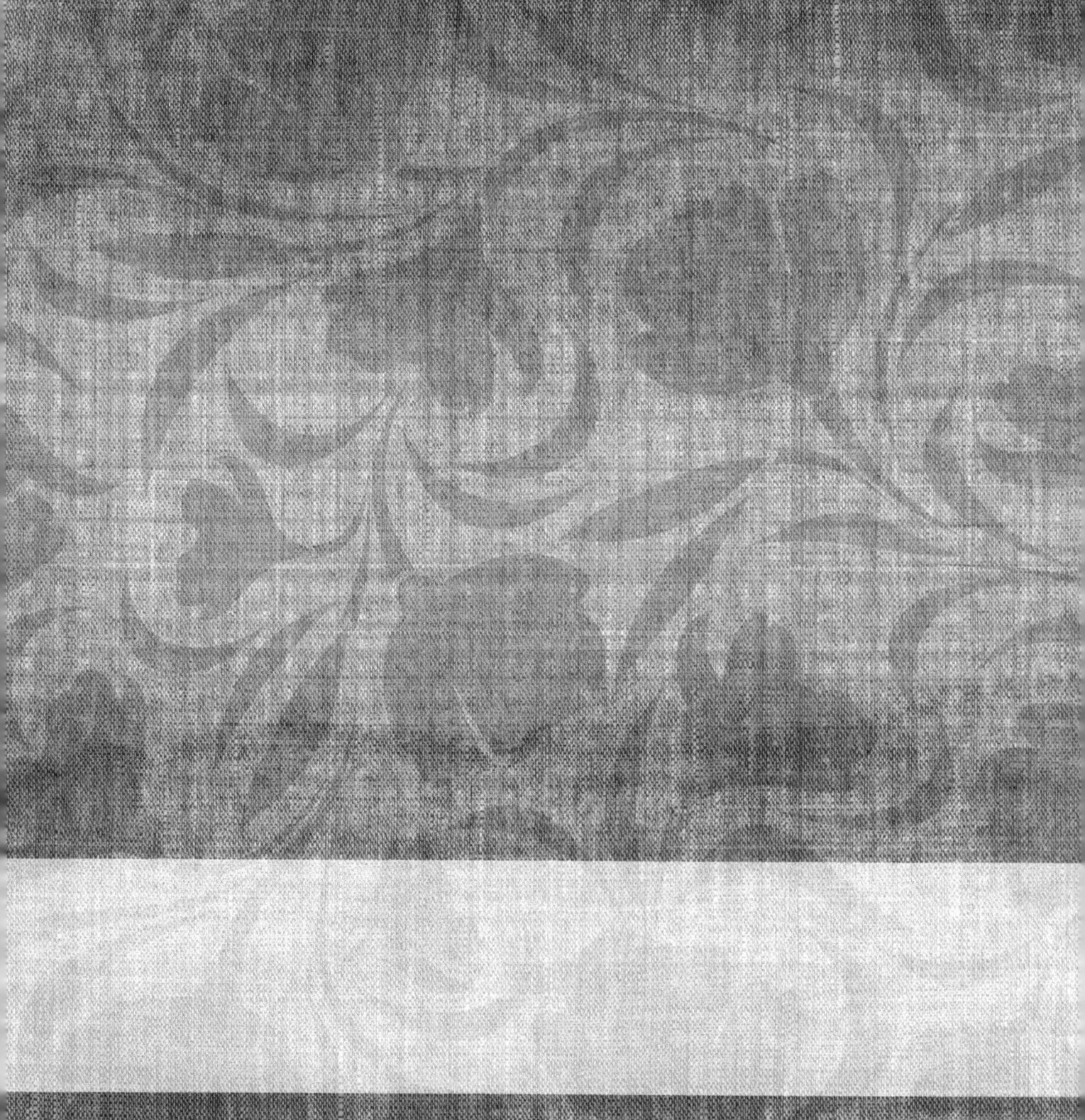

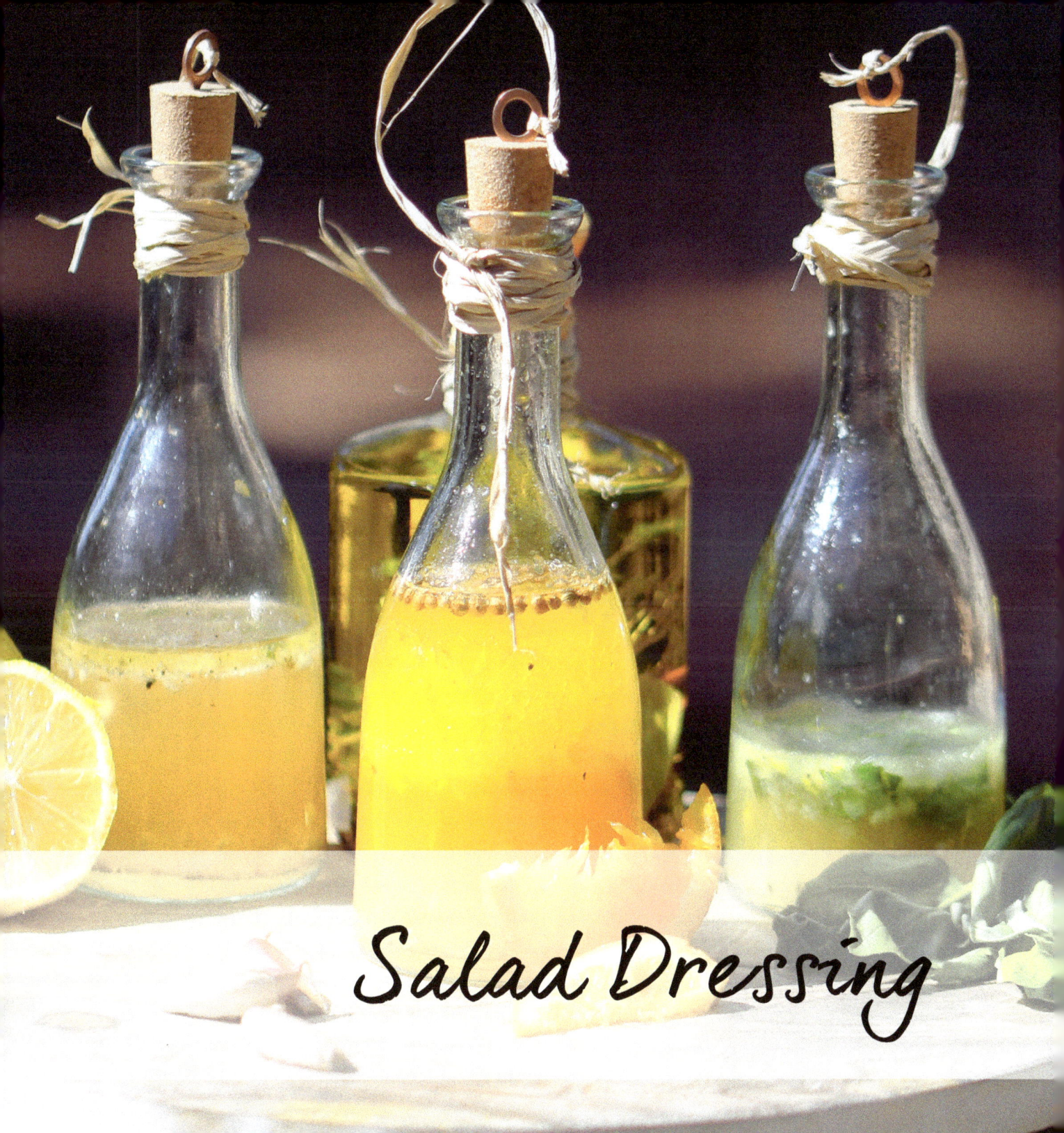

Creamy Capsicum dressing

Ingredients:
1 cup cashews (activated optional)*
½ red capsicum
1 chilli
2 tablespoons nutritional yeast
1 cloves of garlic
1 cup filtered water
Juice of one lemon
A pinch of pink mineral salt

Method:
Place all ingredients into a blender and blend until smooth. Serve with your favorite salads.
*Activated cashews - soaked in salted water for a minimum 2-4 hours then drain.

Mustard-Orange garlic salad dressing

Ingredients:
2 oranges (zest and Juice)
1 teaspoon of spicy mustard seeds
¼ cup of extra light virgin olive oil
Juice of half a lime
Juice of one lemon
1 clove of crushed garlic
Cracked black pepper
1 pinch of pink mineral salt to taste

Method:
Place all ingredients into a glass bottle and shake then serve on your favorite green salad. Best served on the day. You can store in the fridge.

Lemon herb dressing

Ingredients:

Juice of 2 lemons
Zest of one lemon
4-6 leaves fresh oregano
4-6 leaves fresh basil
½ teaspoon of pink mineral salt
Cracked black pepper to taste
1 tablespoon of olive oil
1 teaspoon of coconut sugar (optional)
1 teaspoon of apple cider vinegar

Method:

Finely chop fresh oregano and basil then add to a bowl with other ingredients and mix well. Then store in a glass bottle and serve on your favorite salad as desired.

Apple cider vinegar vinaigrette

Ingredients:

1 clove of crushed garlic
½ teaspoon of mustard seeds crushed
Juice of 1 lime or lemon
1/2 cup organic apple cider vinegar
1 teaspoon raw organic honey
2 dessertspoons extra-virgin olive oil
Pinch of pink mineral salt
Cracked black pepper to taste

Method:

Place all ingredients together in a glass jar and shake well. You are ready to serve.

Spicy tomato sauce

Ingredients:

1kg ripe tomatoes diced
1 cup of sundried tomatoes
2 cups of coconut water or filtered water
2 cloves of crushed garlic
½ red onion diced
2 teaspoons of cumin
6 yellow mustard seeds
1 teaspoon of turmeric powder
2 teaspoons of coconut oil
Juice of one lemon
1 small red chilli or chilli powder (optional)
1 teaspoon olive oil
1 dessertspoon of apple cider vinegar
Pinch of pink mineral salt and pepper to taste

Method:

Place coconut oil into a pot on a medium heat, add onion, garlic, turmeric, chilli and cumin and stir for a few minutes to release aromas and onion is clear. Then place all ingredients from the pot with tomatoes, salt and pepper into a blender and puree. Add pureed mixture back to the pot and simmer for 20 minutes until sauce thickens adding more coconut water if needed. Then remove from heat and allow sauce to cool. Place in airtight glass bottles topped with a spoon of olive oil then seal and store for later use when needed.

Creamy sauté sauce

Ingredients:

1 cup of cashews (activated optional)*
½ cup of brazil nuts
1 spring onion
1 clove of crushed garlic
1 fresh chilli or ground chilli
1 cup of coconut milk or water
1 cm of lemon grass stalk finely sliced
Juice of half a lemon
1 teaspoon of turmeric powder
1 teaspoon of ginger fresh
1 teaspoon of cumin powder
Pink mineral salt to taste
Cracked pepper to taste

Method:

Place all ingredients into blender and blend until smooth. Then add to your favorite salad or use as a marinate on your chicken kebabs.

*Activated cashews - soaked in salted water for a minimum 2-4 hours then drain.

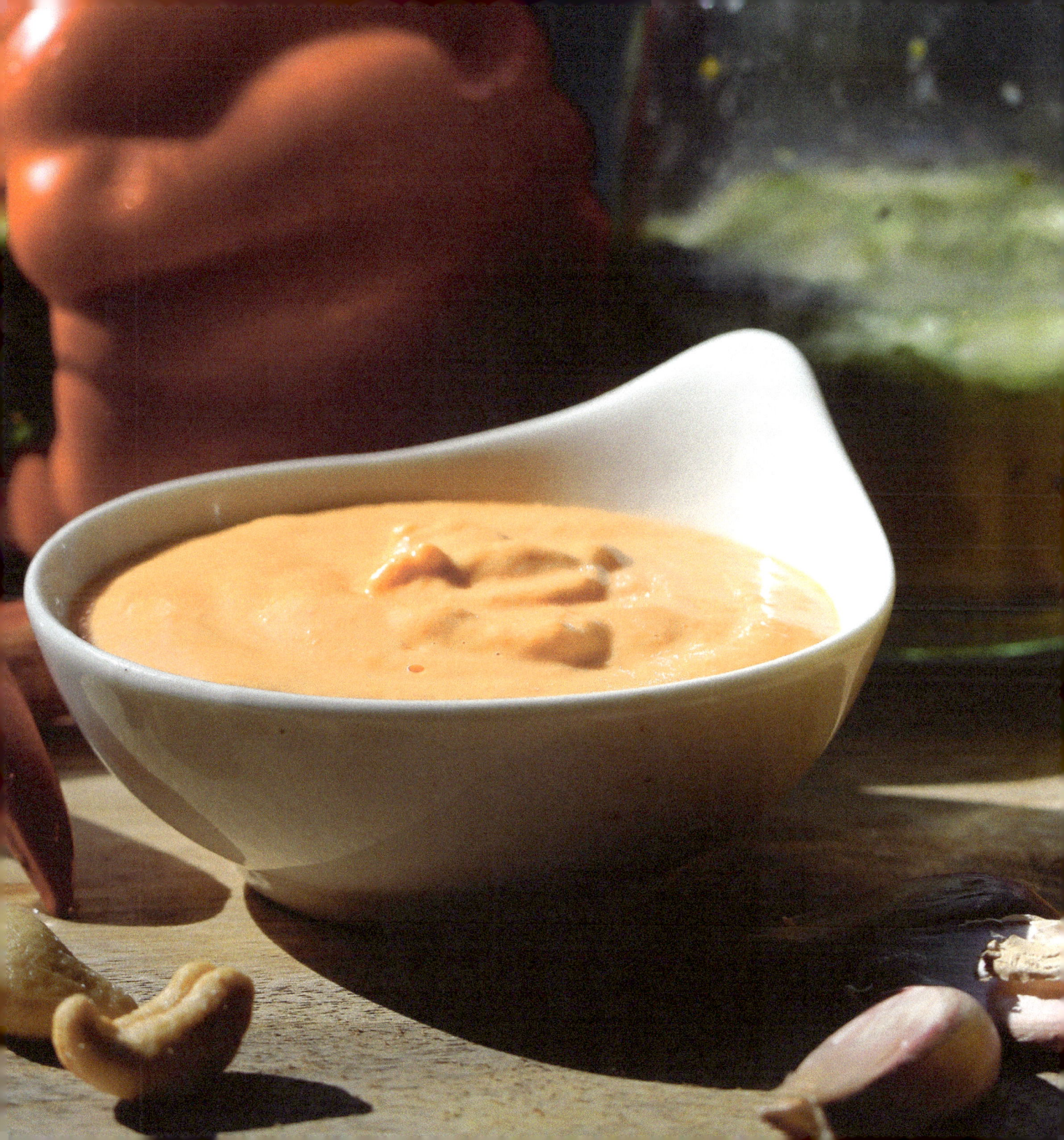

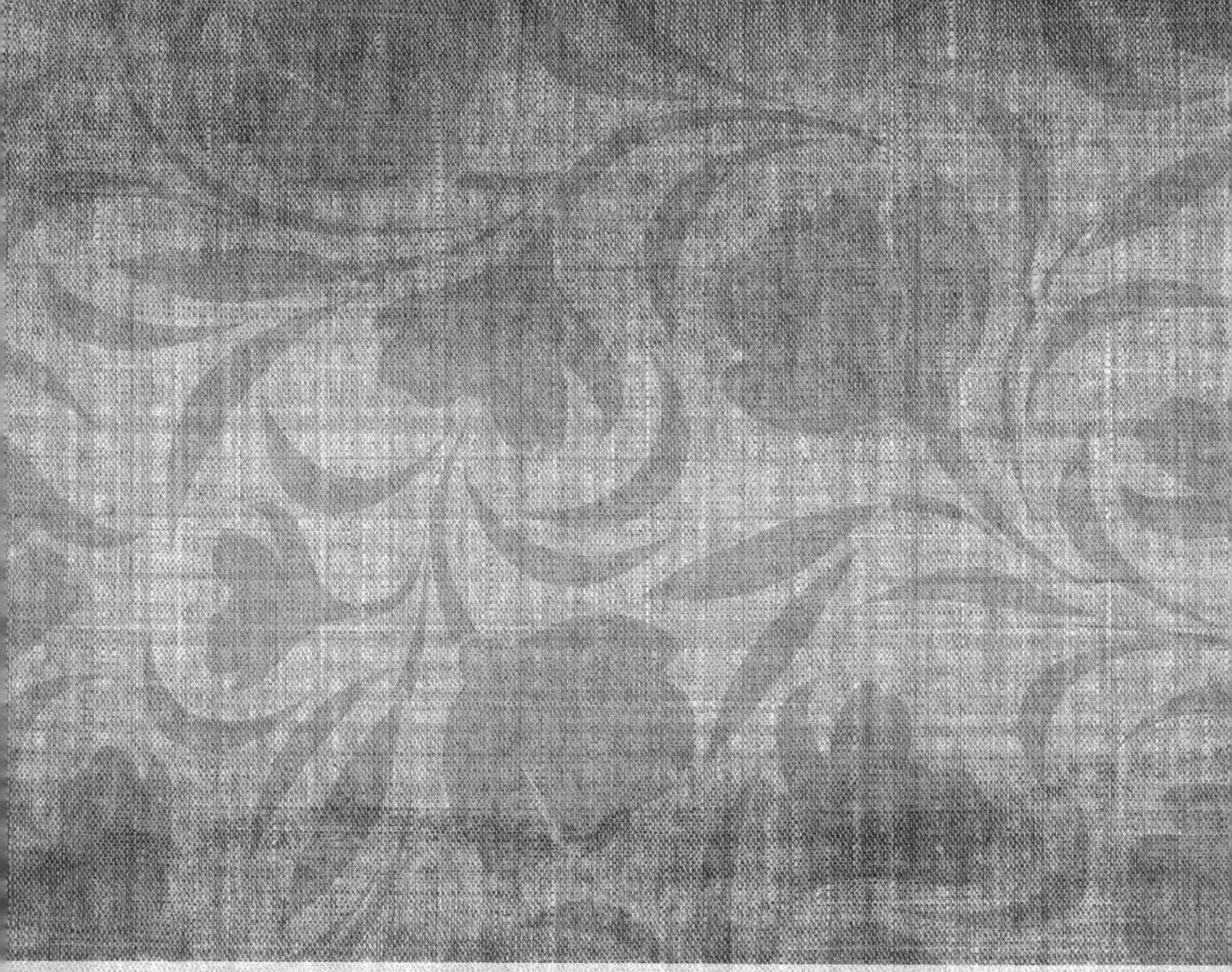

The benefits of fermented foods

Fermented foods contain probiotics which are good bacteria that help keep our gut healthy. This in turn helps keep the immune system in the body healthy. Things that cause a breakdown of the good bacteria in our system range from foods that are processed and contain added sugar, to household chemicals, pollution. There are many benefits to eating fermented foods regularly that contain these probiotics.

*Chisholm D "Have you got the guts to be Really healthy" Australia 2006

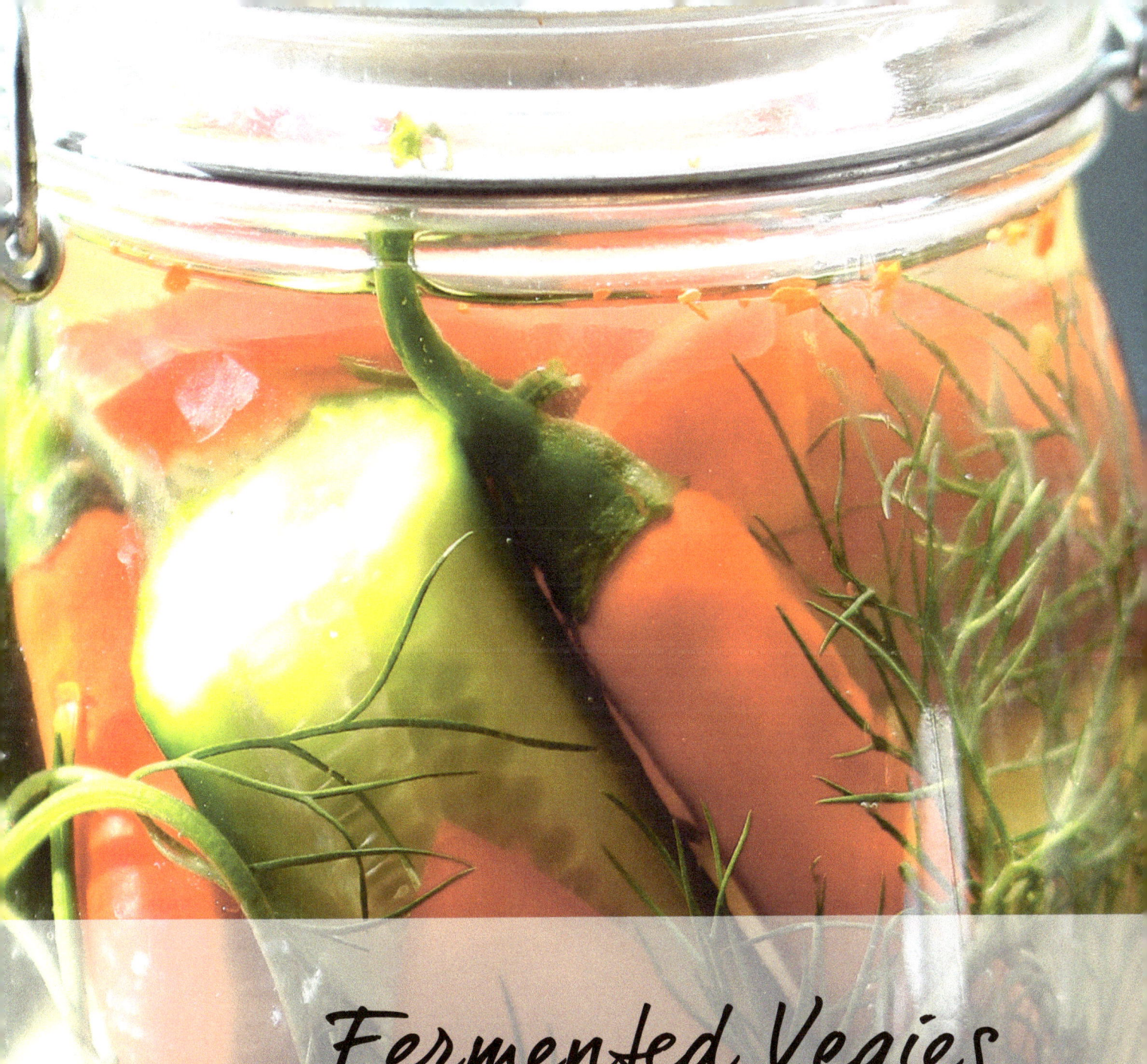

Fermented Vegies

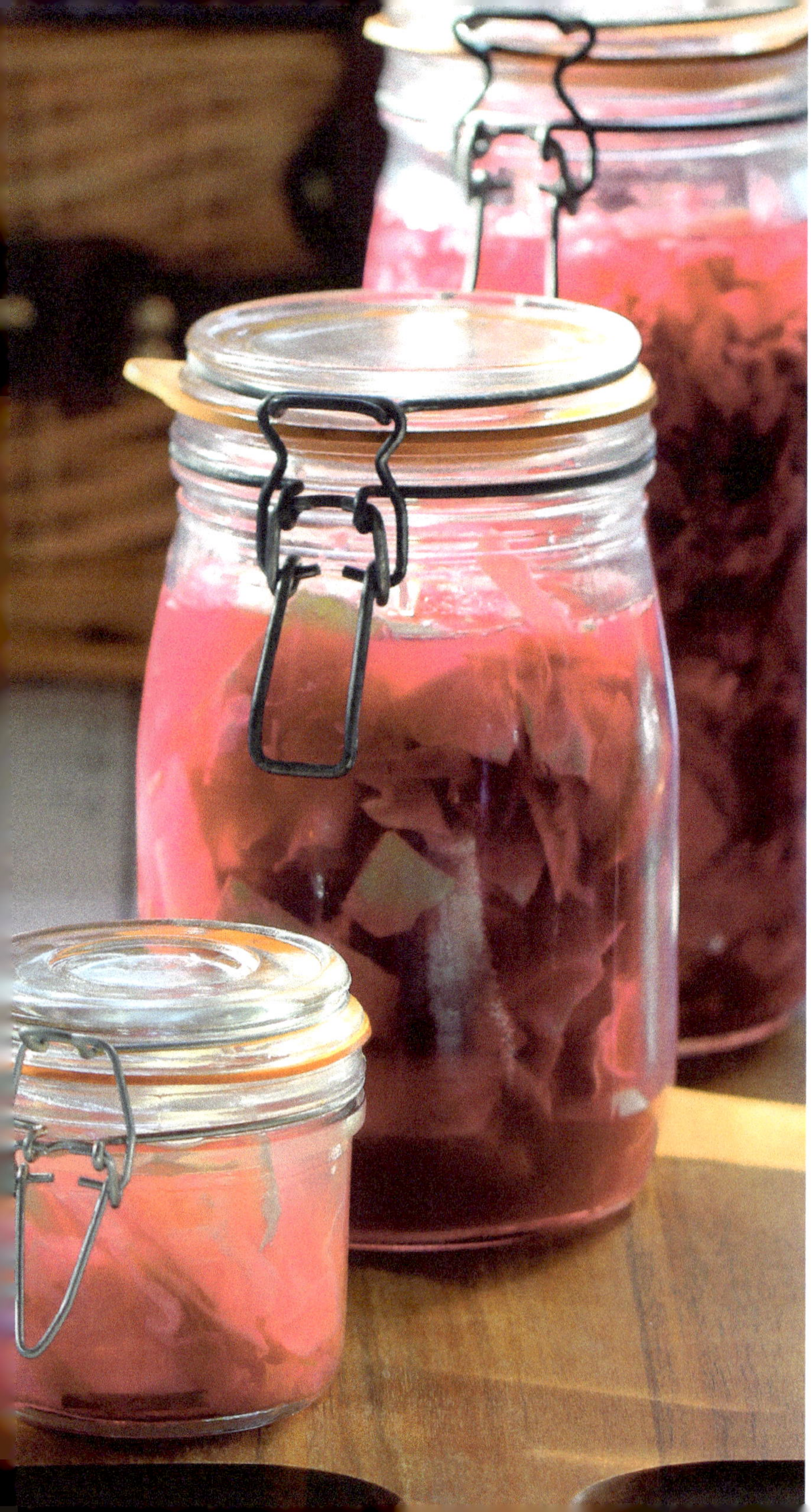

Sauerkraut

Ingredients:
½ a cabbage
Salt (1 teaspoon per cup of water)
Filtered water

Method:
Wash and shred cabbage then place into a 1 litre clean air tight glass jar with filtered water and salt completely dissolved. Make sure the vegetables are completely submerged under the water. Find something to put in the top of the jar to keep them completely submerged. Place on kitchen bench for 6 days out of the sun, then place in the fridge and keep refrigerated. Sauerkraut will last up to 10-12 months in the fridge.

Cucumbers & peppers

Ingredients:

3-4 cucumbers

1 red capsicum sliced

2 red chillies

Dill fresh and seeds

1 clove of garlic

Salt (1 teaspoon per cup of water)

Filtered water to cover the contents

2 tablespoons of liquid from sauerkraut jar

Method:

Wash and place cucumbers and peppers into a 1 litre clean air tight glass jar with filtered water, 1 teaspoon of salt per cup of water. Make sure the vegetables are completely submerged under the water. Find something to put in the top of the jar to keep them completely submerged. It is important that they remain under the liquid for the whole duration of the fermenting process. You want to avoid mold developing and ruining your batch.

Place on kitchen bench for 6 days out of the sun, then refrigerate. If you prefer vinegary taste add a couple of tablespoons of apple cider vinegar to the jar and leave for another week.

Fermented coconut cream

Ingredients:

1 can of full fat coconut milk or cream

1 sachet of Kefir cultures*

Method:

Blend coconut milk and contents of Kefir sachet cultures. Then Place mixture into a 1 litre airtight glass jar and store in a cool, dark corner on your kitchen bench out of direct sunlight for 24 hours swirling periodically. The creamy coconut drink is ready to serve. Keep refrigerated, will last up to one week when kept in the fridge.

Note: Buy kefir cultures suitable for coconut derivatives.

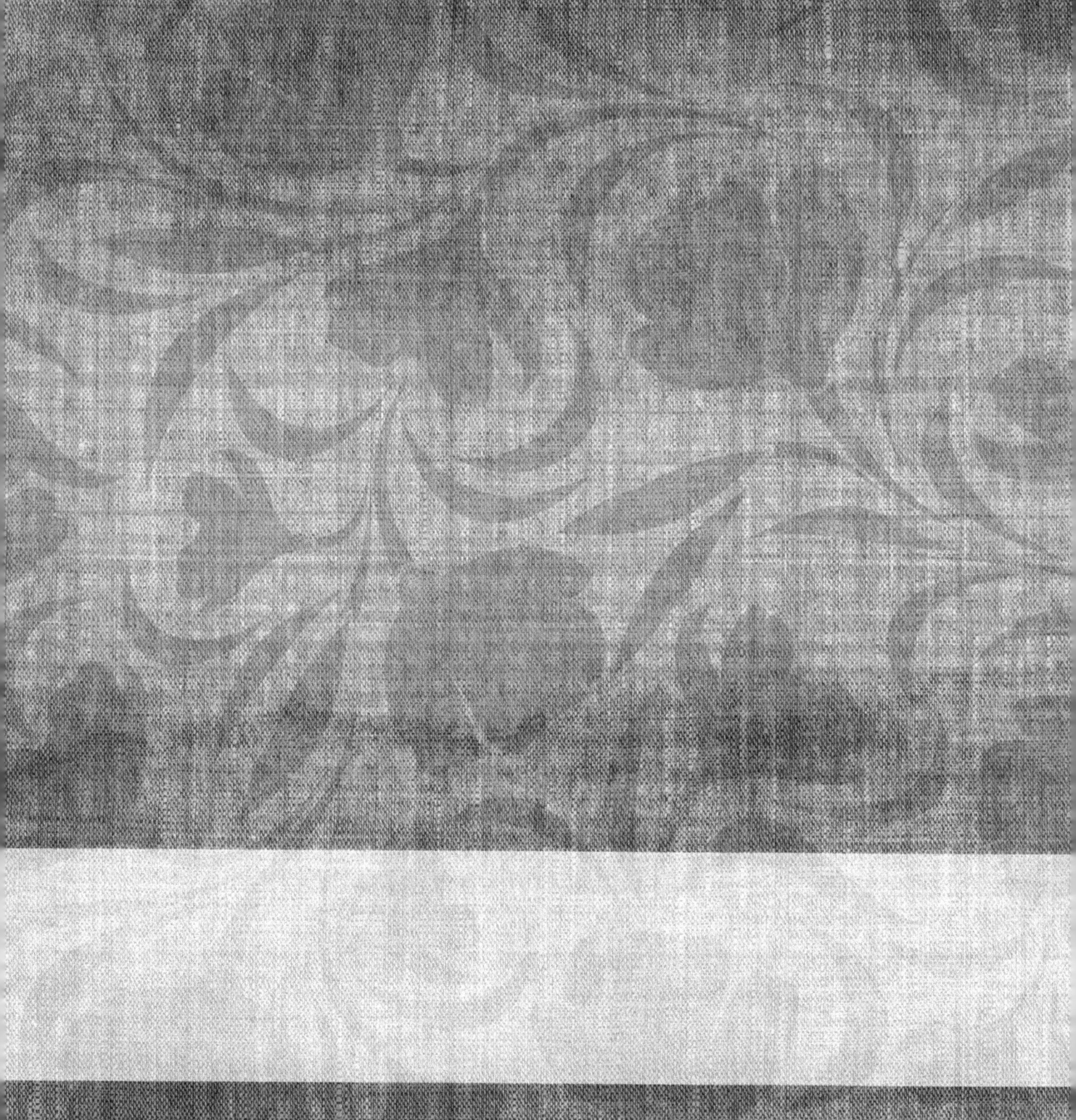

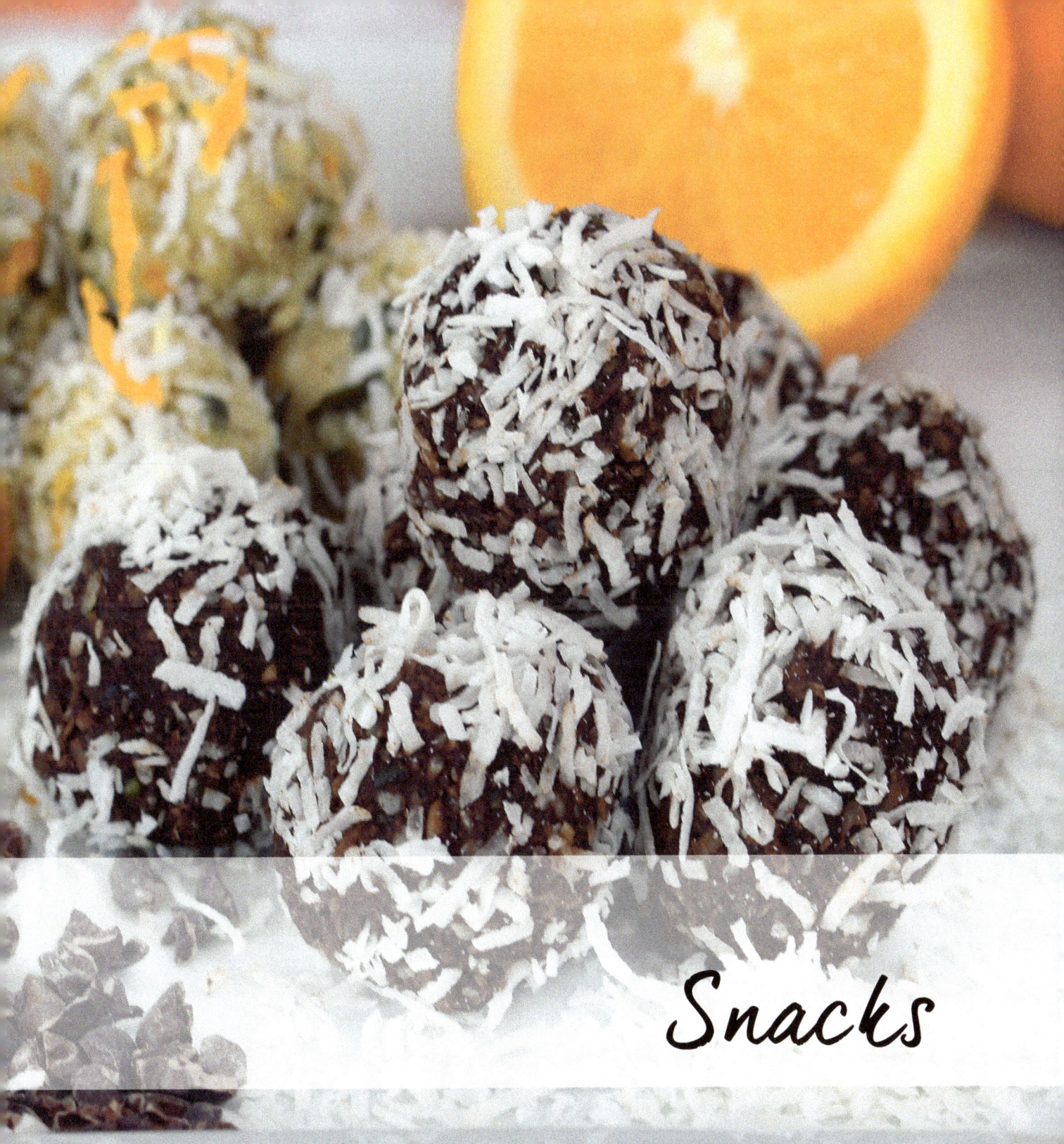

Snacks

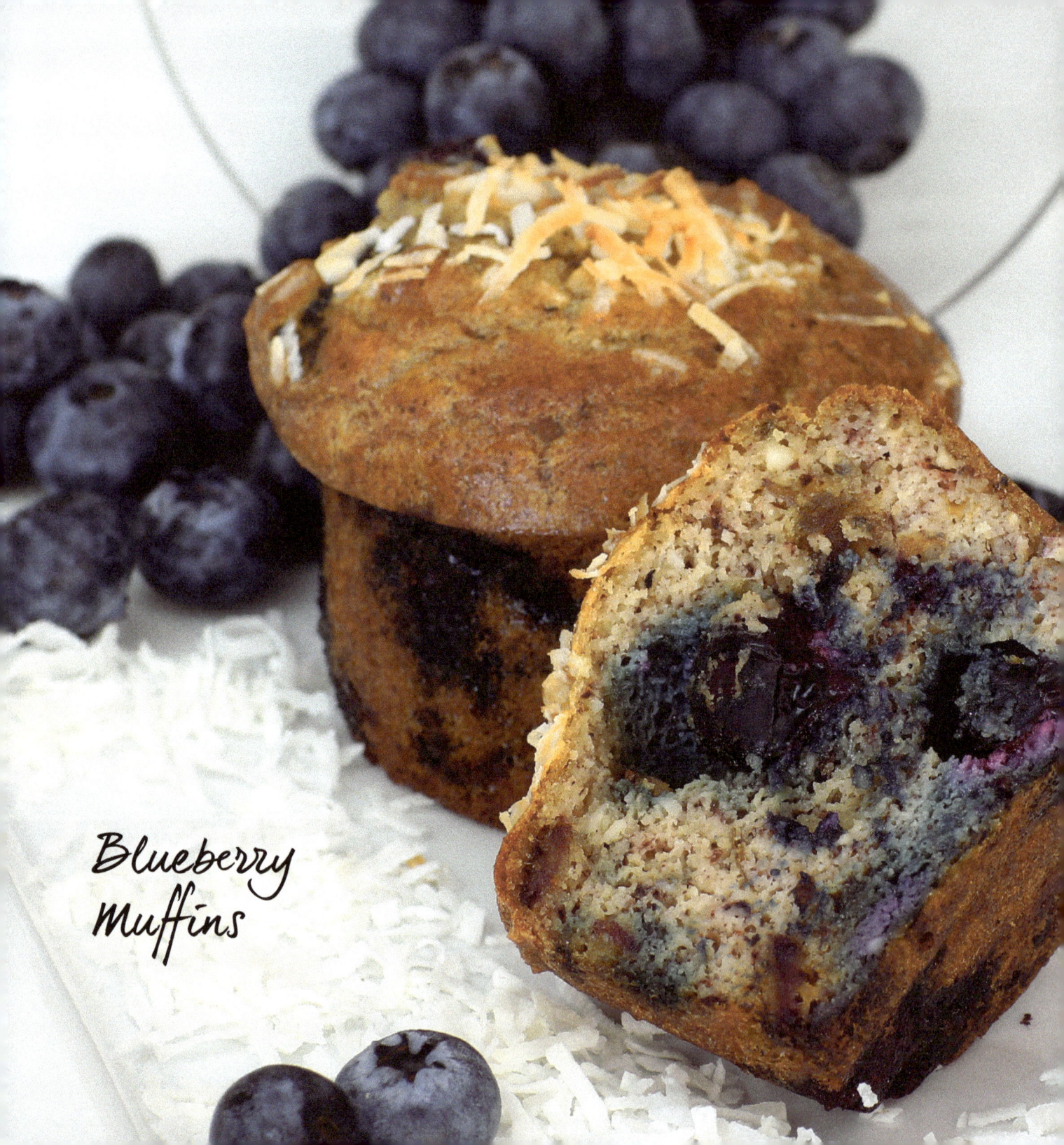
Blueberry Muffins

Chocolate chia muffins

Ingredients: makes 8-9 muffins

1 cup of almond meal

1/2 cup of hazelnut meal (almond meal can be used)

I teaspoon of chia seeds

4 organic eggs

1 teaspoon of bi-carb soda

10-15 dates (chopped finely)

1 teaspoon of vanilla extract

1+half teaspoon of raw organic cacao powder

¼ cup of coconut oil

¾ cup of filtered hot water to soften dates

Shredded coconut as topping

½ teaspoon of pink mineral salt

Method:

Preheat oven to 175degrees- fan forced 165degrees. Place finely chopped dates into a small bowl in hot water to soak. Place all dry ingredients into large glass bowl and add eggs and vanilla extract mix for 30 seconds. Then add dates, water and coconut oil and mix well.

Place mixture into muffin trays and sprinkle with shredded coconut. Bake for 18-20 minutes. Place on cooling rack. Once room temp place in airtight container and put in the fridge.

Blueberry muffins

Ingredients: makes 8-9 muffins

1 & half cups of almond or hazelnut meal (or half of each)

1 teaspoon of chia seeds (optional)

4 organic eggs

1 teaspoon of bi-carb soda

10-15 dates (chopped finely)

1 teaspoon of vanilla extract (optional)

1 cup of fresh blueberries (optional diced apple)

¼ cup of coconut oil

¾ cup of filtered boiled hot water to soften dates

Method:

Preheat oven to 175degrees- fan forced 165degrees. Place dates into a small bowl in hot water to soak. Place all dry ingredients into large glass bowl and add eggs and vanilla extract mix for 30 seconds. Then add dates, water and coconut oil and mix well. Finally gently fold blueberries into mixture.

Place mixture into muffin trays and sprinkle with shredded coconut. Bake for 18-20 minutes. Place on cooling rack. Once room temp place in airtight container and put in the fridge.

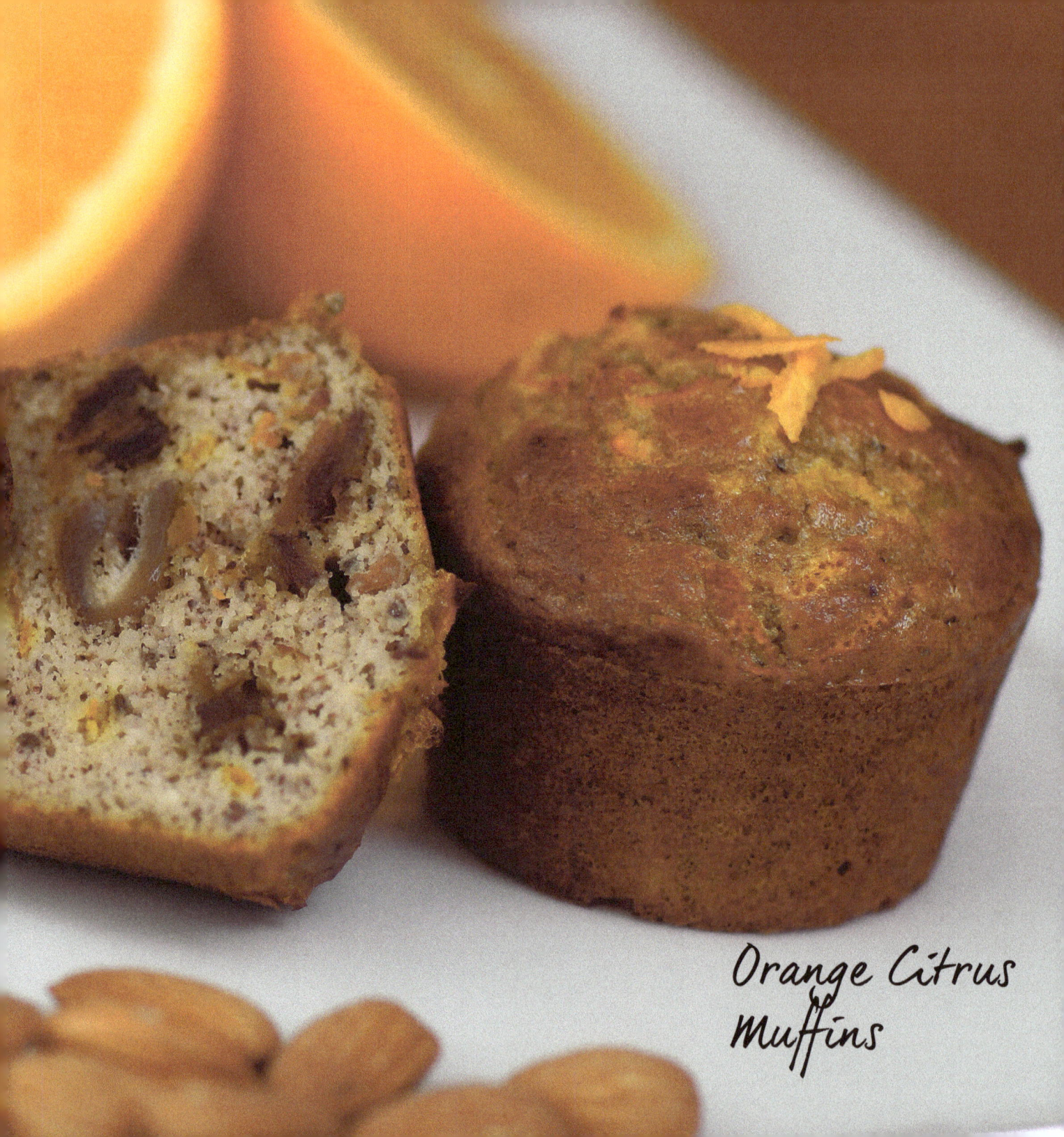

Orange Citrus Muffins

Orange citrus muffins

Ingredients: makes 8-9 muffins

2 cups of almond meal
I teaspoon of chia seeds
5 organic free range eggs
1 teaspoon of bi-carb soda
1 cup of dates (chopped finely)
½ cup of fresh orange juice
2 dessertspoons of orange zest
Juice of 1 lime
¼ cup of coconut oil
1 teaspoon of vanilla extract (optional)
Filtered hot water to soften dates

Method:
Preheat oven to 175 degrees- fan forced 165 degrees. Place dates into a small bowl in hot water to soak. Place all dry ingredients into large glass bowl and add eggs and vanilla extract mix for 30 seconds. Then add drained dates, lime juice, orange juice, orange zest, and coconut oil and mix well.
Place mixture into muffin trays. Bake for 18-20 minutes. Place on cooling rack. Once room temp place in airtight container and put in the fridge.

Savory slice & muffins

Ingredients: makes 9-10 muffins

1 grated carrot
3 grated zucchini
1 cup baby spinach leaves chopped
1 onion diced and cooked in a little coconut oil (optional)
Half a red capsicum diced
4-5 eggs
1 & half cups of almond meal or 1 cup of coconut flour
¼ cup of coconut oil
1teaspoon of bi-carb soda
Pinch of pink mineral salt, cracked black pepper and sprinkle of powdered chilli

Method:
Pre heated oven 175-180 degrees Celsius. Place all ingredients into a glass bowl and mix well with a fork. Place into oven proof dish and place into the oven for 25-30 minutes. Serve Hot or Place on cooling tray for 30 minutes and then into air tight container in the fridge. A great midmorning snack.
Muffins
Place mixture into muffin tray and bake for 20-25 minutes. Test to see if cooked by placing a skewer in the center of each muffin. If it comes out clean the muffins are cooked. Time may vary depending on your oven.

Raw orange cake-balls

Ingredients: makes 20 -25 balls

1 cup of blanched almond meal

1 cup of hazelnut meal

¼ cup of pepitas (pumpkin) seeds chopped fine

¼ cup of pine nuts

¼ cup of hazel nuts chopped

1/3 cup of organic coconut oil

Zest of two oranges

Juice of two oranges

Juice of one lime

1 teaspoon of ground cinnamon

1 dessertspoon of organic honey or coconut sugar

I cup of shredded coconut

Method:

Mix all dry ingredients together well in a glass bowl then add orange and lime juice and finally coconut oil. Mix well to combine together. Spoon out a heaped teaspoon size of mixture and roll in shredded coconut. Place balls in airtight container in the fridge. Berry Juice can be substituted for orange juice for a change. These make an ideal snack for in between meals.

For cake; place mixture into a deep ceramic cake mold pressing mixture firmly into place. Refrigerate for 2-3 hours. Turn upside down and remove from mold. Top with shredded coconut, Fruit of your choice - berries or orange wedges go well. Blend berries of your choice with a little lemon juice and honey added, then drizzle over cake.

Note: Use coconut sugar in place of honey to suit Vegan diets.

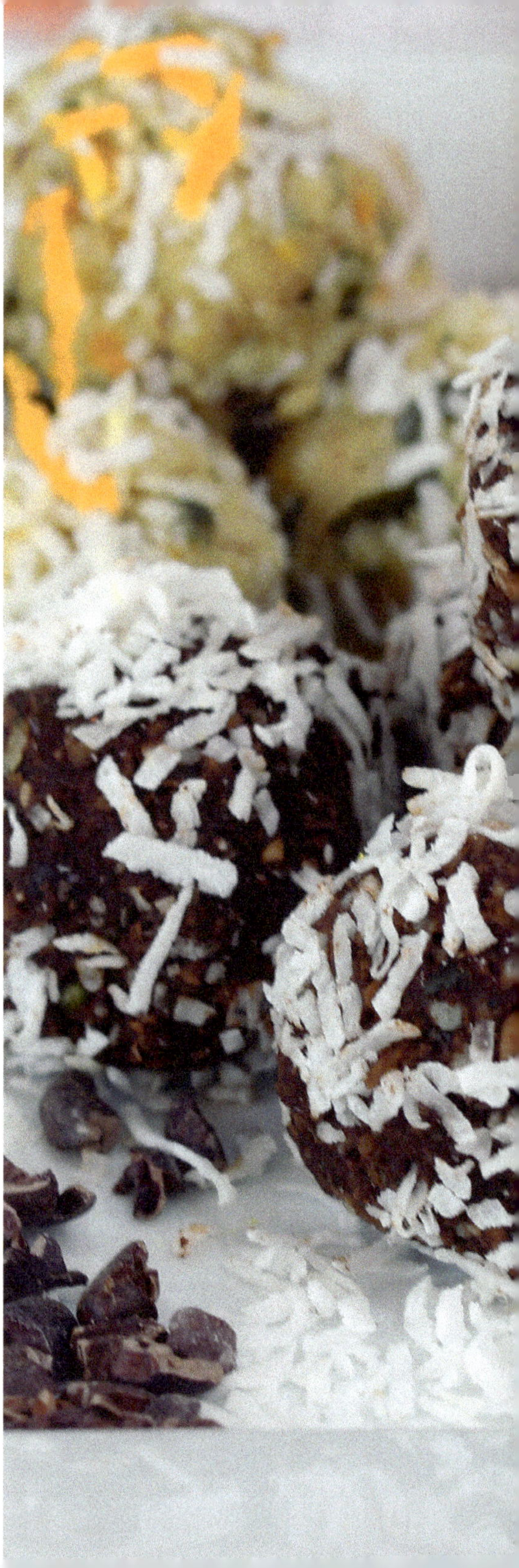

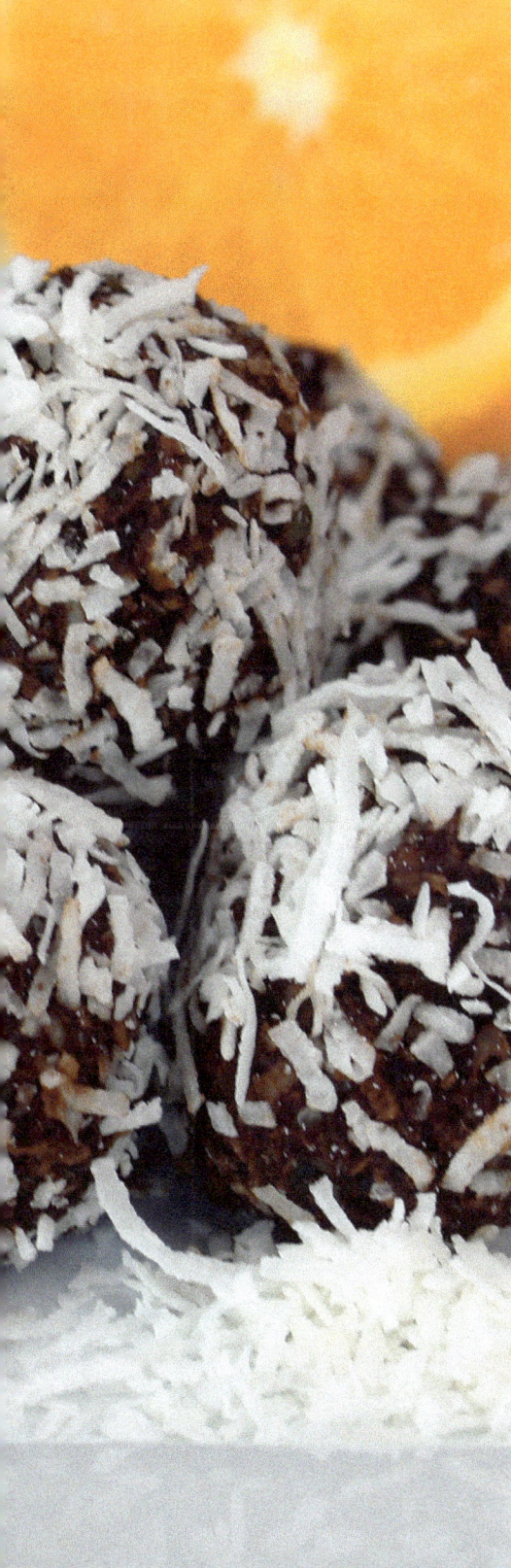

Raw chocolate balls

Ingredients: 20 balls (depending on the size)

1 cup of almond meal
1 cup of hazelnut meal
1/2 cup of pepitas (pumpkin) seeds
1/2 cup of sunflower seeds
1 cup of shredded coconut (extra for coating balls)
4 tablespoons of chia seeds
4 table spoons of sesame seeds
½ cup of organic cacao powder
Pinch of pink mineral salt
1 cup of dates (softened in hot water)
¾ cup of orange juice
1 dessertspoon of coconut oil

Method:

Place nuts into food processor and pulse to a fine meal and place in a bowl, then add all other dry ingredients and mix with fork. Mix dates well into paste by adding orange juice then add to dry mixture. Stir in coconut oil mix well. Spoon out a heaped teaspoon size of mixture and roll in shredded coconut. Place in fridge in airtight container. Berry Juice can be substituted for orange juice for a change. These make an Ideal snack for in between meals.

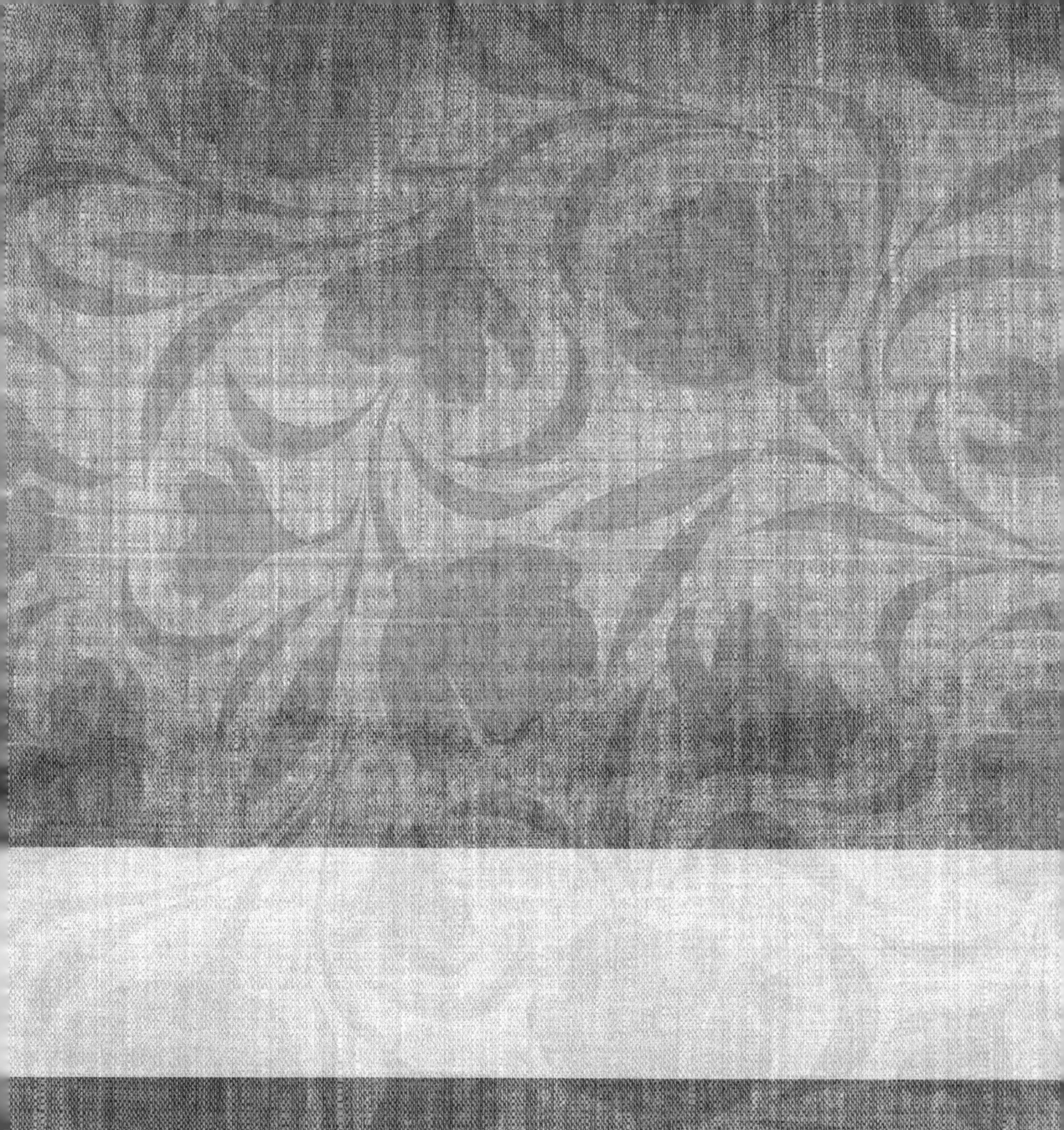

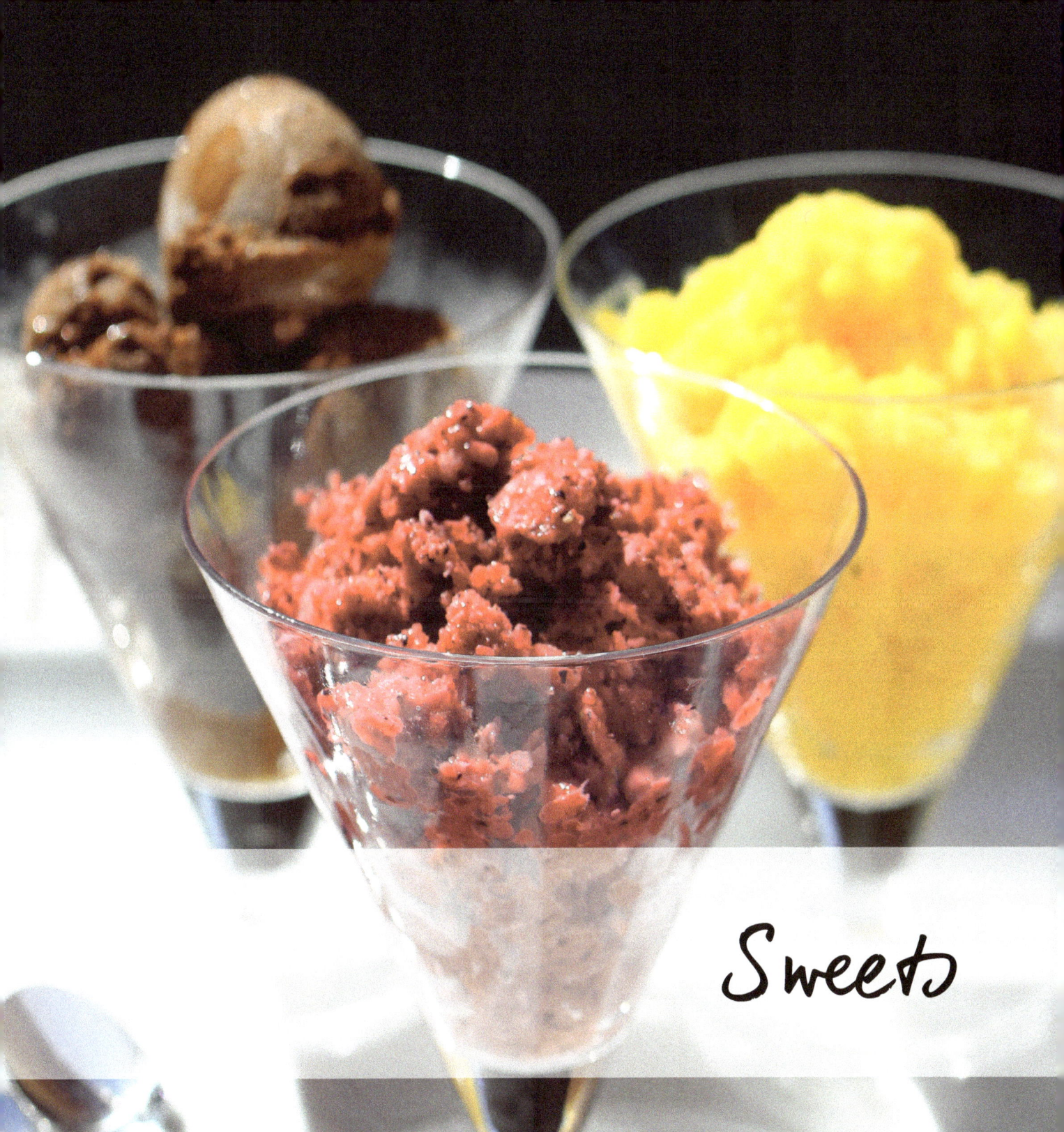
Sweets

Berry Coconut Chocolate

Ingredients:

½ cup raw organic cacao powder
1/4 cup organic coconut oil
1/4 cup of coconut butter or cacao butter
1-2 teaspoons of raw organic honey
One cup of mixed berries (cherries, blueberries, raspberries)
One teaspoon of vanilla extract
¼ cup of shredded coconut

Method:

Place the coconut butter and oil into a small bowl or cup then place the small bowl inside a large bowl of hot water to melt. Once mixture is over 18 degrees it turns to liquid.

Or alternatively place in a bowl on top of a saucepan with 5cm/2inches of water on low heat, when coconut oil and butter melt remove from heat and mix in cacao powder, add honey, essence and finally berry mix, shredded coconut and place onto flat tray lined with foil or baking paper. Place in the fridge to set. Break up into small pieces ready for serving, store in airtight container in the fridge. Alternatively pour mixture into chocolate molds and place in fridge once hard turn out of molds and store in airtight container in the fridge.

Almond Nut Chocolate

Ingredients:

½ cup raw organic cacao powder
1/4 cup organic coconut oil
1/4 cup of coconut butter or cacao butter
1-2 teaspoon of raw organic honey or coconut sugar
½ cup of chopped almonds or mixed nuts
Pinch of Pink mineral salt

Method:

Gently heat coconut butter and oil in a cup by putting the cup or small bowl on top of a saucepan with 10cm/ 2inches of water and place on low heat to melt once over 18 degrees it turns to liquid.

Then mix oil, butter and cacao powder in a bowl add honey and nut mix and place onto flat tray lined with foil or baking paper. Place in the freezer to set around 15 minutes. Break up into small pieces ready for serving, store in airtight container in the fridge.

Chocolate coated fruit

Ingredients:

½ cup organic cocoa
1/4 cup organic coconut oil
1/4 cup of coconut butter or cacao butter
1-2 teaspoons of raw organic honey or ¼ cup of coconut sugar
Fruit in season strawberries, mandarin, cherries
¼ cup of shredded coconut
½ teaspoon of vanilla extract (optional)
Crushed almonds or chia seeds for coating (optional)

Method:

Place coconut butter and oil in a small bowl and place on top of a pot gently heat into a large bowl of hot water to melt once over 18 degrees it turns to liquid remove from heat. Then add cacao powder, honey and essence in with the melted coconut mixture. Then dip fruit into chocolate and roll in shredded coconut or crushed almonds and place onto flat tray lined with foil. Place in the freezer to set around 15 minutes. Then serve otherwise store in airtight container in the fridge.

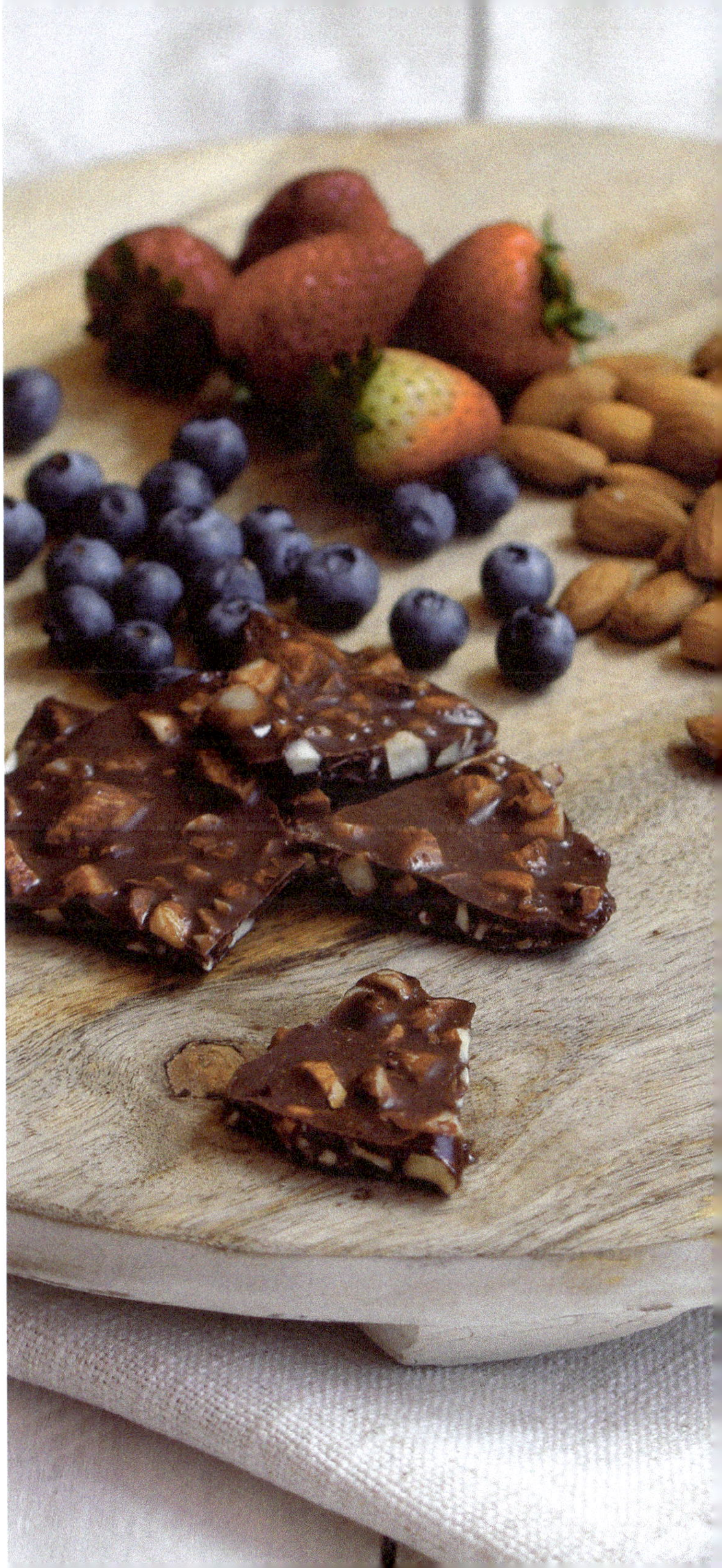

Berry coconut frozen gelato

Ingredients: 8-10 serves
2 cup of strawberries
½ cup of raspberries or blue berries
1 cup of coconut milk or cream
Squeeze of lemon
¼ cup of shredded coconut
1 teaspoon of coconut sugar (optional)

Method:
Place all ingredients into a blender or food processor and blend until smooth. Scoop into BPA free icy polo molds or freezer safe container and freeze for several hours until firm. Icy polls are an idea snack or after dinner treat. The frozen gelato can be scooped into glass bowls and served with extra berries and a sprig of mint.

Berry Fruit topping
Ingredients:
2 cups of mixed berries
½ cup coconut water
1 teaspoon of organic honey (optional) or coconut sugar (vegan)
Juice of ½ lime

Method:
Place ingredients into blender and blend until you have smooth syrup, adding a little more coconut water if needed. Serve on top on cakes and gelato.

Mango/pine fruit gelato

Ingredients: 8-10 serves
2 cups of fresh pineapple
1 cup of mango
1 orange (zest + juice)
Juice of one lemon
1 cup of coconut milk

Method:
Place all ingredients into a blender or food processor and blend until smooth. Scoop into BPA free icy polo molds or freezer safe container and freeze for several hours until firm. Icy polls are an idea snack or after dinner treat. The frozen gelato can be scooped into glass bowls and served with chopped nuts and shredded coconut.

Mocha gelato

Ingredients: 2-4 serves
¼ cup of raw organic cacao powder
1 dessertspoon of coffee powder
1 cup of coconut Cream
½ cup of coconut water
1 dessertspoon of raw organic honey or coconut sugar (vegan option)

Method:
Place all ingredients into a blender or food processor and blend until smooth. Scoop into BPA free icy polo molds or freezer safe container and freeze for several hours until firm. Icy polls are an idea snack or after dinner treat. The frozen gelato can be scooped into glass bowls and served with Cacao nibs or coffee granules.

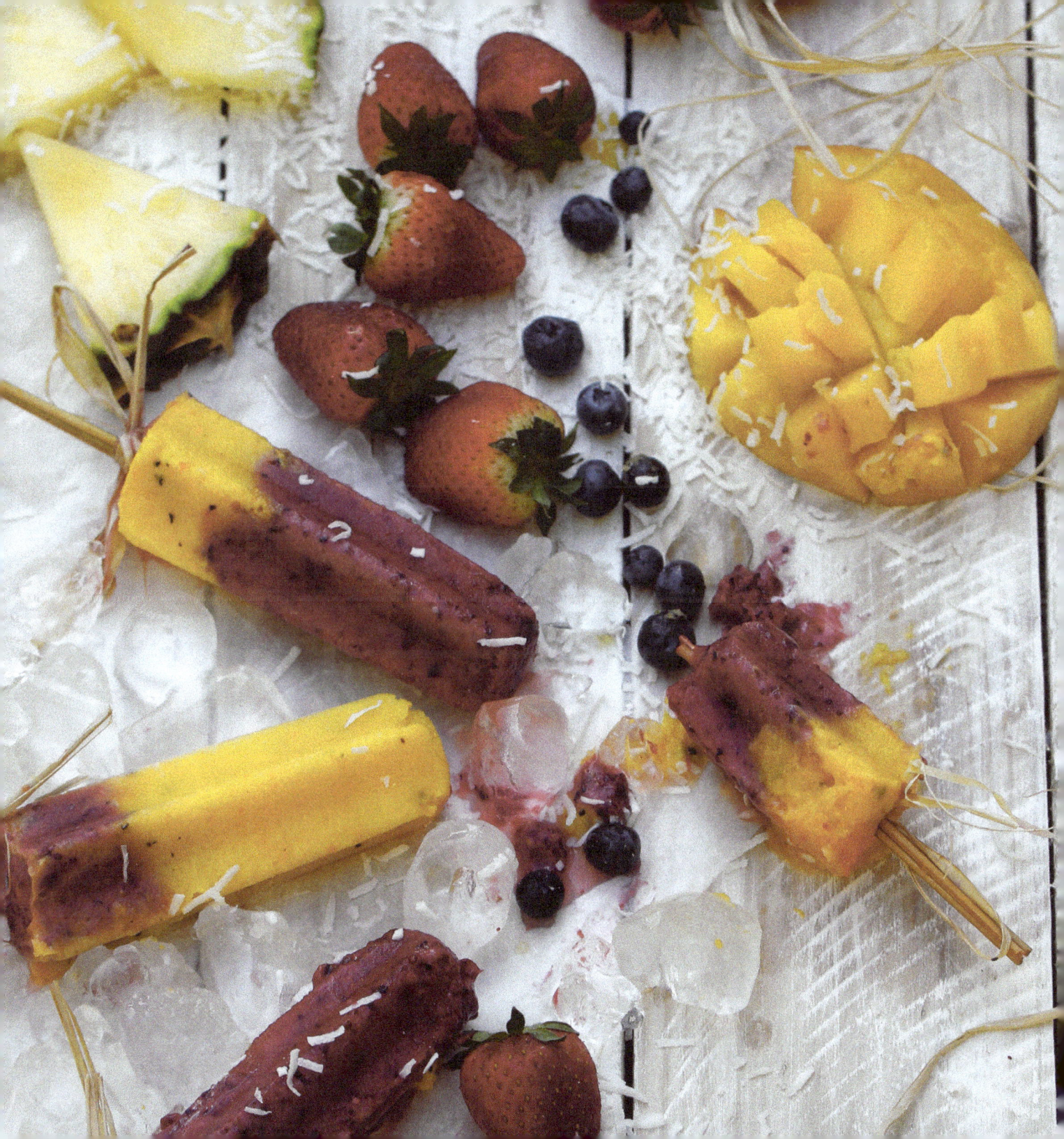

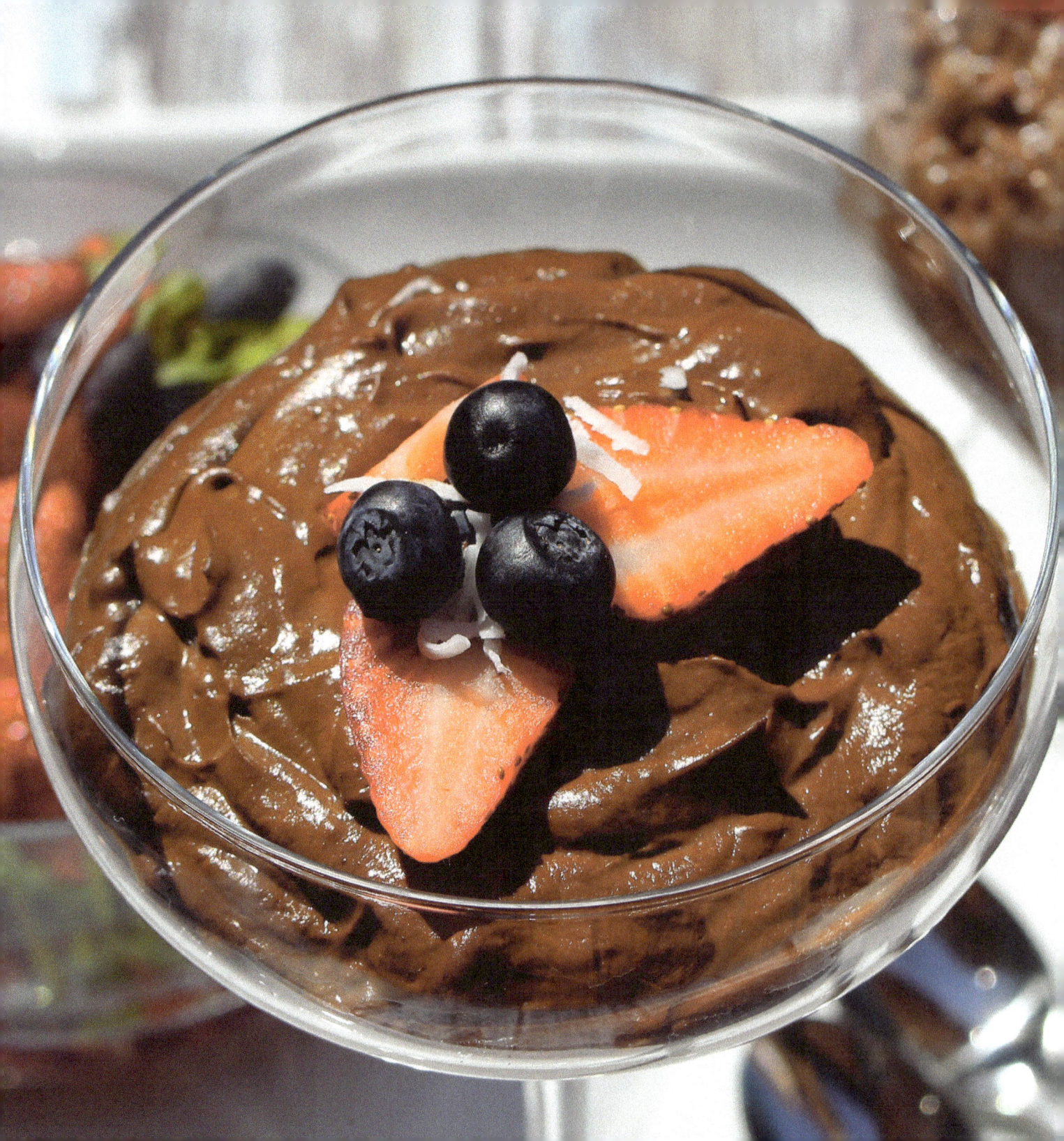

Chocolate mousse

Ingredients: 4-6 serves

1 banana
1 avocado
½ cup of raw cacao powder
1 cup of coconut cream
2 teaspoons of raw organic honey or coconut sugar (vegan option)

Method:

Place all ingredients into a blender and blend until smooth. Place into small desert bowl or glass and place in fridge to chill, then top with a sprinkle of shredded coconut or crushed cashew nuts and serve. Another option for dinner parties place berries or fruit of your choice into parfait glass and top with mousse mixture and refrigerate to chill, top with berries and crushed cashews.

Chia vanilla pudding

Ingredients: 2-4 serves

½ cup chia seeds
2 cups coconut milk
1 vanilla stick fresh
(1 teaspoon optional vanilla extract)
1/2 teaspoon of cinnamon
2 teaspoons of coconut sugar (optional)
1 tablespoon of raw cacao powder
(as a chocolate option)

Method:

Mix all ingredients together in a glass bowl and refrigerate for 2 hours or until ingredients are set. Chocolate option: add 2 dessertspoons of organic cacao powder to make a chocolate pudding.
Fruit puréed can also be used as an alternative flavour.

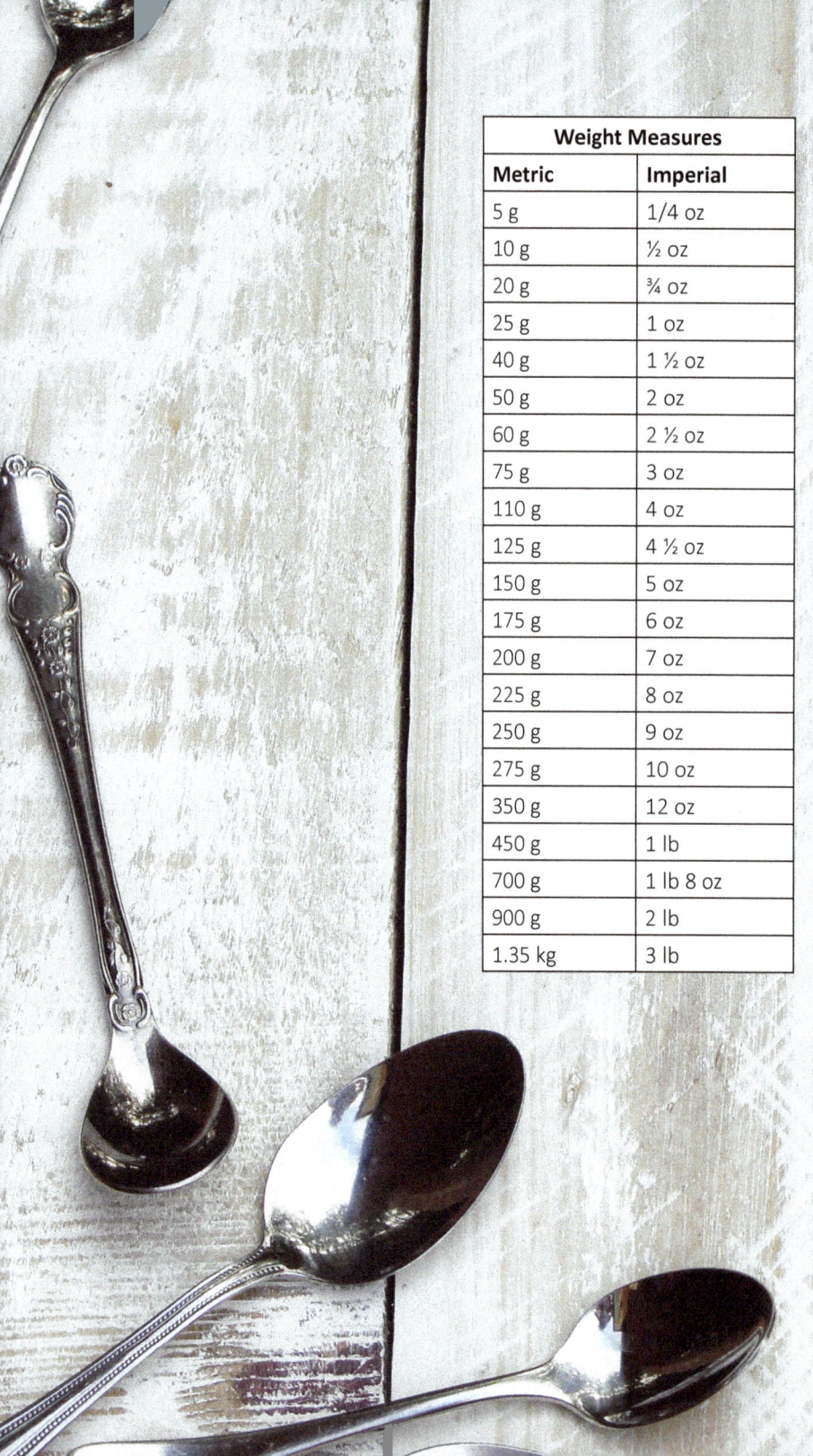

Weight Measures	
Metric	Imperial
5 g	1/4 oz
10 g	½ oz
20 g	¾ oz
25 g	1 oz
40 g	1 ½ oz
50 g	2 oz
60 g	2 ½ oz
75 g	3 oz
110 g	4 oz
125 g	4 ½ oz
150 g	5 oz
175 g	6 oz
200 g	7 oz
225 g	8 oz
250 g	9 oz
275 g	10 oz
350 g	12 oz
450 g	1 lb
700 g	1 lb 8 oz
900 g	2 lb
1.35 kg	3 lb

Volume Measures	
Metric	Imperial
1.25 ml	1/4 tsp
2.5 ml	1/2 tsp
5 ml	1 tsp
10 ml	2 tsp
15 ml	1 tbsp/ 4 tsp
30 ml	2 tbsp
45 ml	3 tbsp
60 ml	4 tbsp
75 ml	5 tbsp
90 ml	6 tbsp
15 ml	1/2 fl oz
30 ml	1 fl oz
50 ml	2 fl oz
75 ml	3 fl oz
100 ml	3.5 fl oz
125 ml	4 fl oz
150 ml	5 fl oz
175 ml	6 fl oz
200 ml	7 fl oz
225 ml	8 fl oz
250 ml	9 fl oz
275 ml	10 fl oz
400 ml	14 fl oz
500 ml	18 fl oz
570 ml	1 pint
725 ml	1 ¼ pint
1 litre	1 ¾ pint

tsp = teaspoon   tbsp = tablespoon

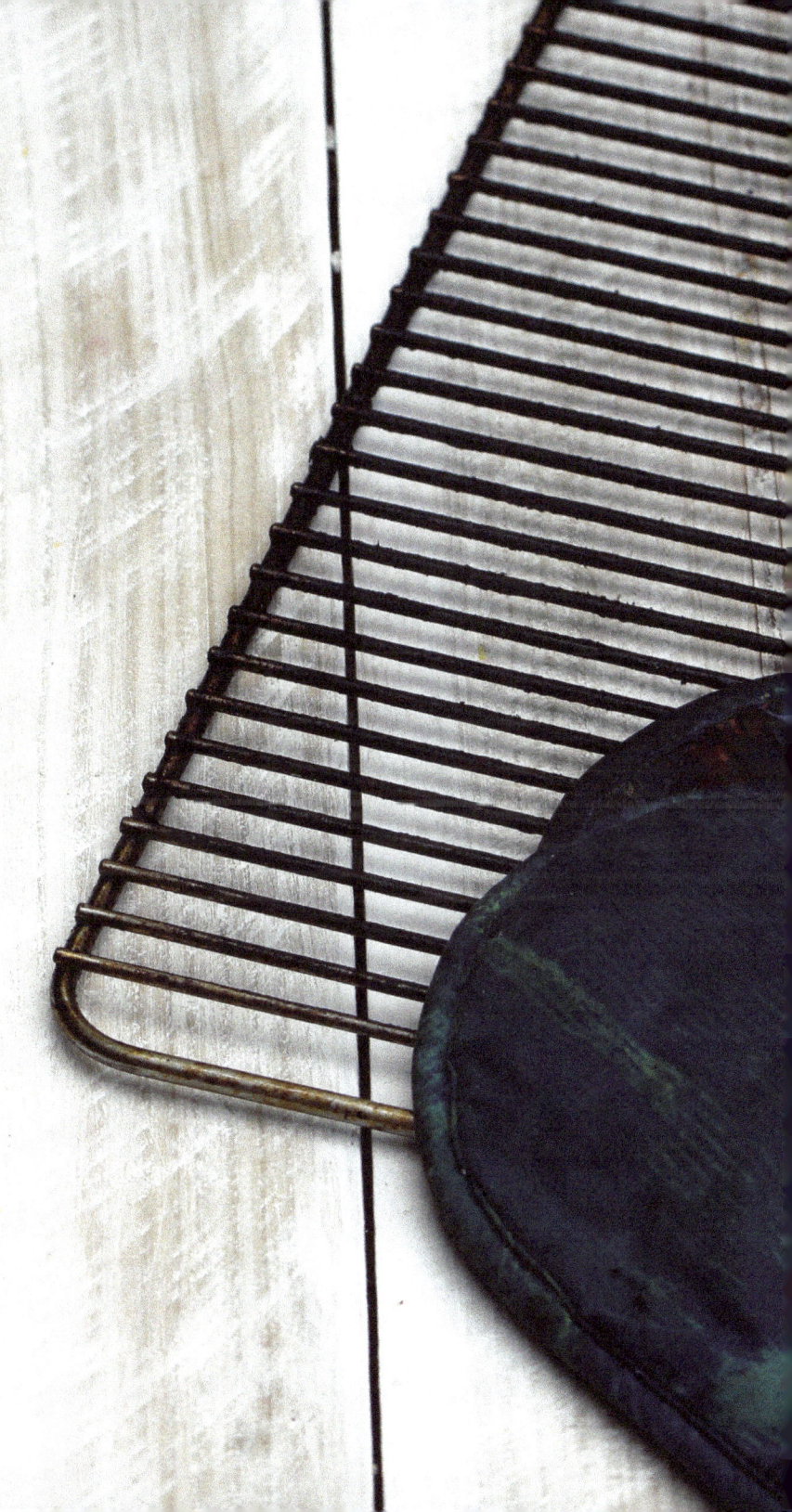

Liquid Convesions		
Metric	Imperial	spoon/cup
15 ml	½ fl oz	1 tbsp
30 ml	1 fl oz	1/8 cup
60 ml	2 fl oz	¼ cup
120 ml	4 fl oz	½ cup
240 ml	8 fl oz	1 cup

Oven Temperatures		
°F	°C	Gas
275°F	140°C	1
300°F	150°C	2
325°F	170°C	3
350°F	180°C	4
375°F	190°C	5
400°F	200°C	6
425°F	220°C	7
450°F	230°C	8
475°F	240°C	9

If not using a fan forced oven, you will need to increase the oven temperature in a recipe by 10 degrees.

References

Websites

Alkaline vs acid chart. http://www.acidalkalinediet.com/Alkaline-Foods-Chart.htm
AROC Values. 2010.http://oracvalues.com
Coconut Research Center. 2010.www.coconutresearchcenter.org
Nuts and seeds nutritional information http://www.nutrition-and-you.com
Wikipedia, the free encyclopedia http://en.wikipedia.org/wiki
Review effects of dietary fibre and its components on
metabolic health * Nutrients 2010 James M. Lattimer and Mark D. Haub www.mdpi.com/journals/nutrients

Books

Batmanghlidj,F MD. And Phillip Day. The Essential Guide to Water and Salt. Kent, Great Britain; Credence Publications, 2008

Clum, Dr. Lauren and Mariza Snyder. The Antioxidant Counter. Berkley,CA: Ulysses Press' 2011.

Chisholm D "Have you got the guts to be Really healthy" Australia 2006

Fife, Bruce N.D., Foreword by Conrado S. Dayrit, M.D Coconut Cures. Piccadilly Books,2005

Fife, Bruce and, Jon J. Kabara The Coconut Oil Miracle. Avery Trade.2004

Wolfe, David. Superfoods; The Food and Medicine of the future. Berkley, CA; North Atlantic Books, 2009.

Resource Guide

Power Superfoods
Specializes in organic superfoods
Find the following here:
Acai powder, cacao powder and nibs, chia seeds,
goji berries, maca powder, Peruvian pinch of pink
mineral salt, maqui powder
Visit: www.powersuperfoods.com

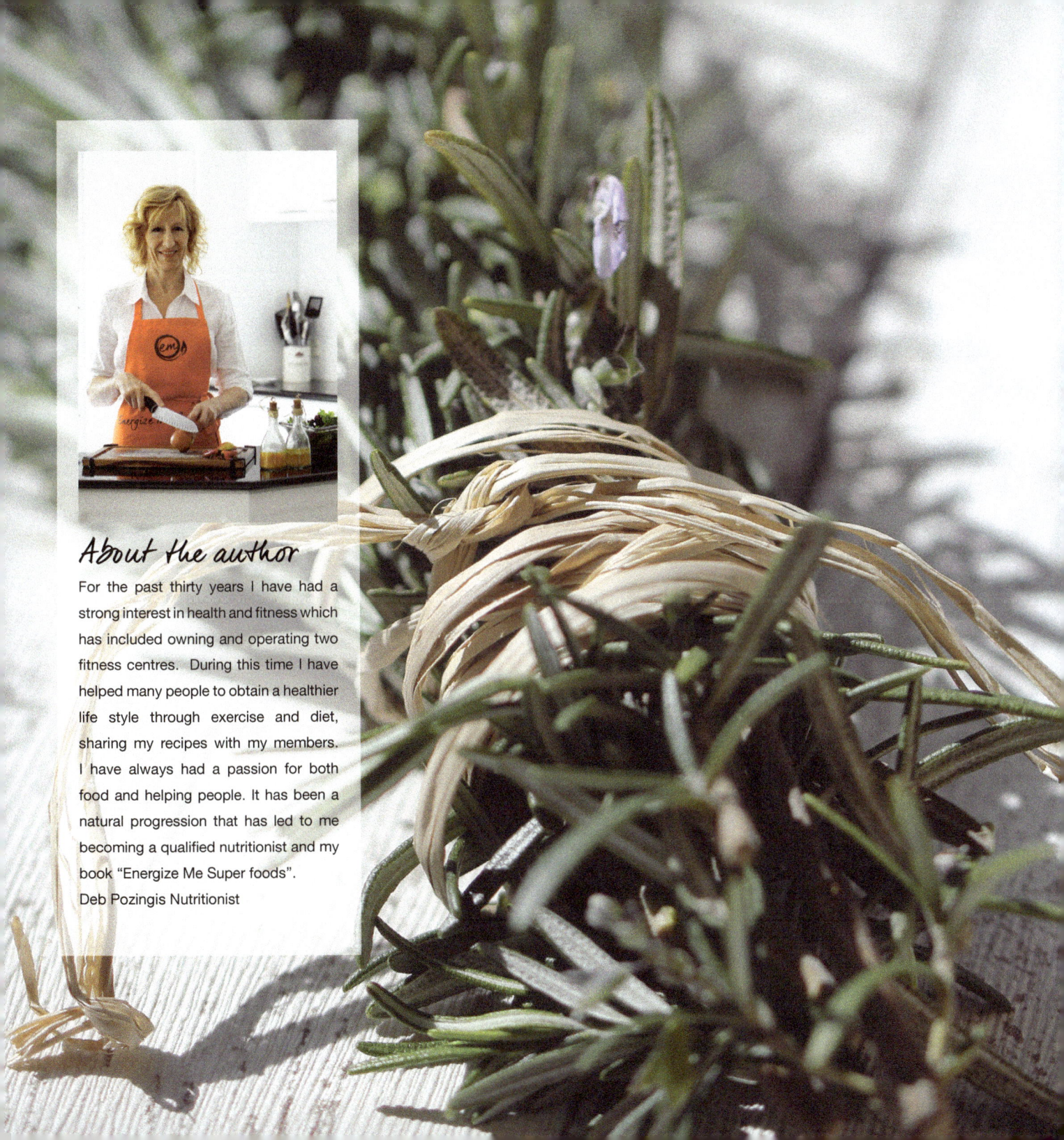

About the author

For the past thirty years I have had a strong interest in health and fitness which has included owning and operating two fitness centres. During this time I have helped many people to obtain a healthier life style through exercise and diet, sharing my recipes with my members. I have always had a passion for both food and helping people. It has been a natural progression that has led to me becoming a qualified nutritionist and my book "Energize Me Super foods".

Deb Pozingis Nutritionist

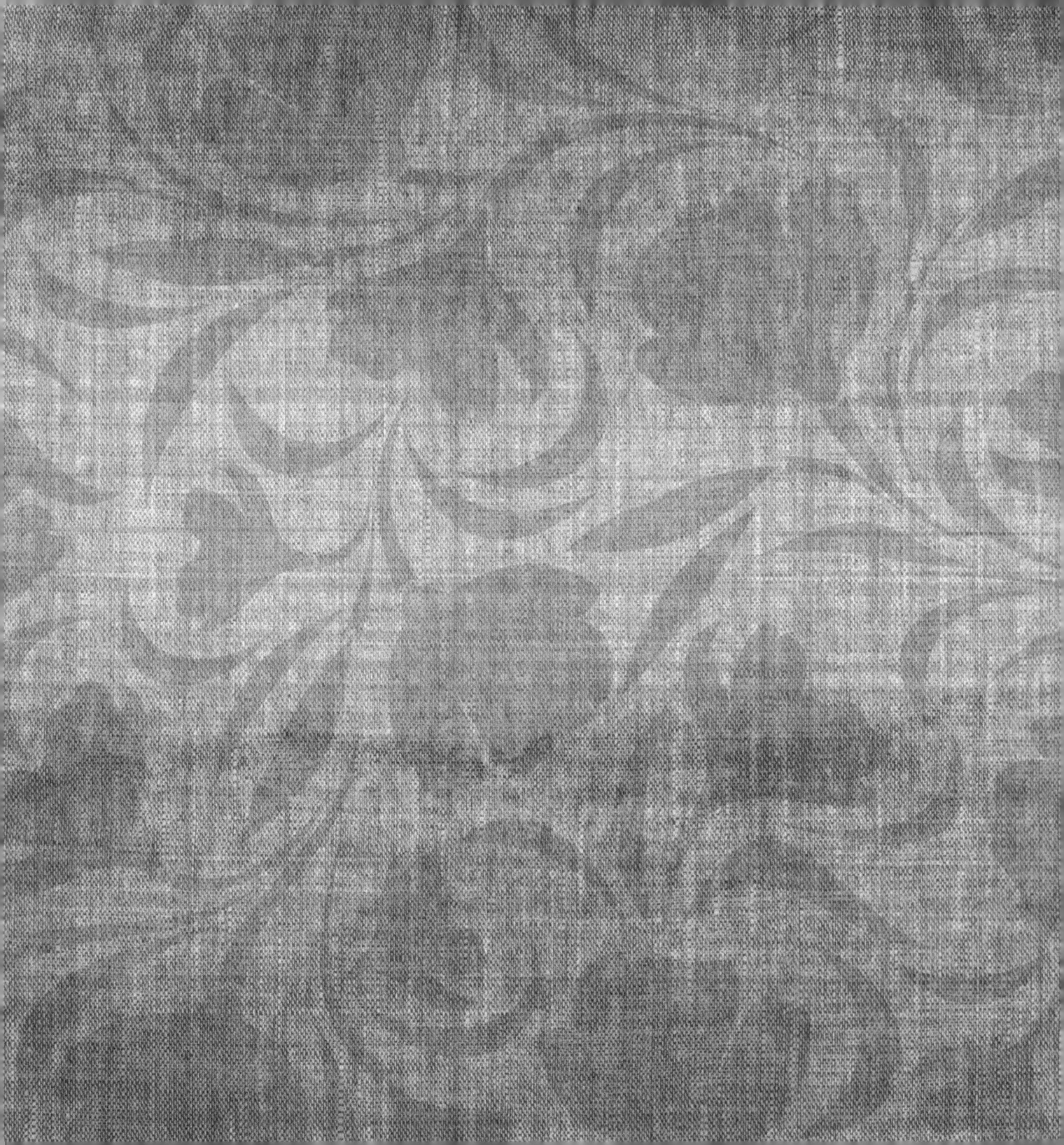

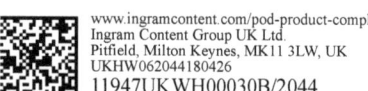

www.ingramcontent.com/pod-product-compliance
Ingram Content Group UK Ltd.
Pitfield, Milton Keynes, MK11 3LW, UK
UKHW062044180426
11947UKWH00030B/2044

9 780994 159700